before2

HOW TO EAT WELL AND LOSE WEIGHT

Diana Frangi & Silvia Branca

Published by Red Box Publishing. U.K.
Editor: Sherron Mayes from The Editing Den
Book design: Gabriela Koppel : : : www.frilans.es

ISBN 978-1-5272-8528-6

acknowledgements

We would like to express our deepest gratitude for the invaluable contribution and inspiring support from our dear friends, Sherron Mayes, Yael Breuer, Glen Whittaker and Lofty Lawrence who all helped bring this book to life.

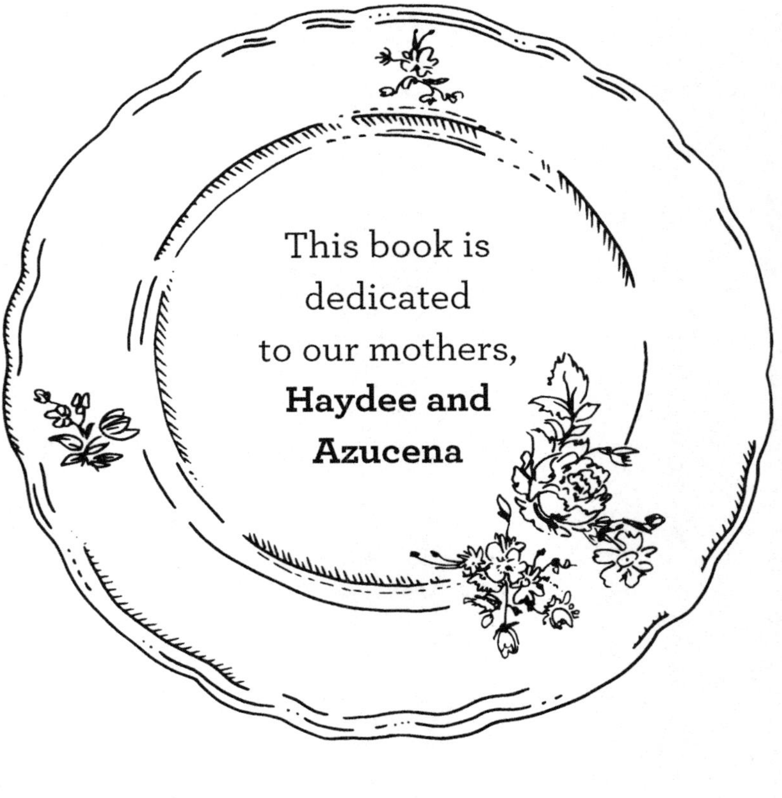

This book is
dedicated
to our mothers,
Haydee and
Azucena

a note to the reader

The material in this book is designed to provide helpful information on the Before 2 eating plan. It is not intended as a substitute for medical advice. For diagnosis or treatment of any health issues, consult your doctor or physician. The authors and publisher are not accountable for the use or application of any of the information contained in this book.

contents

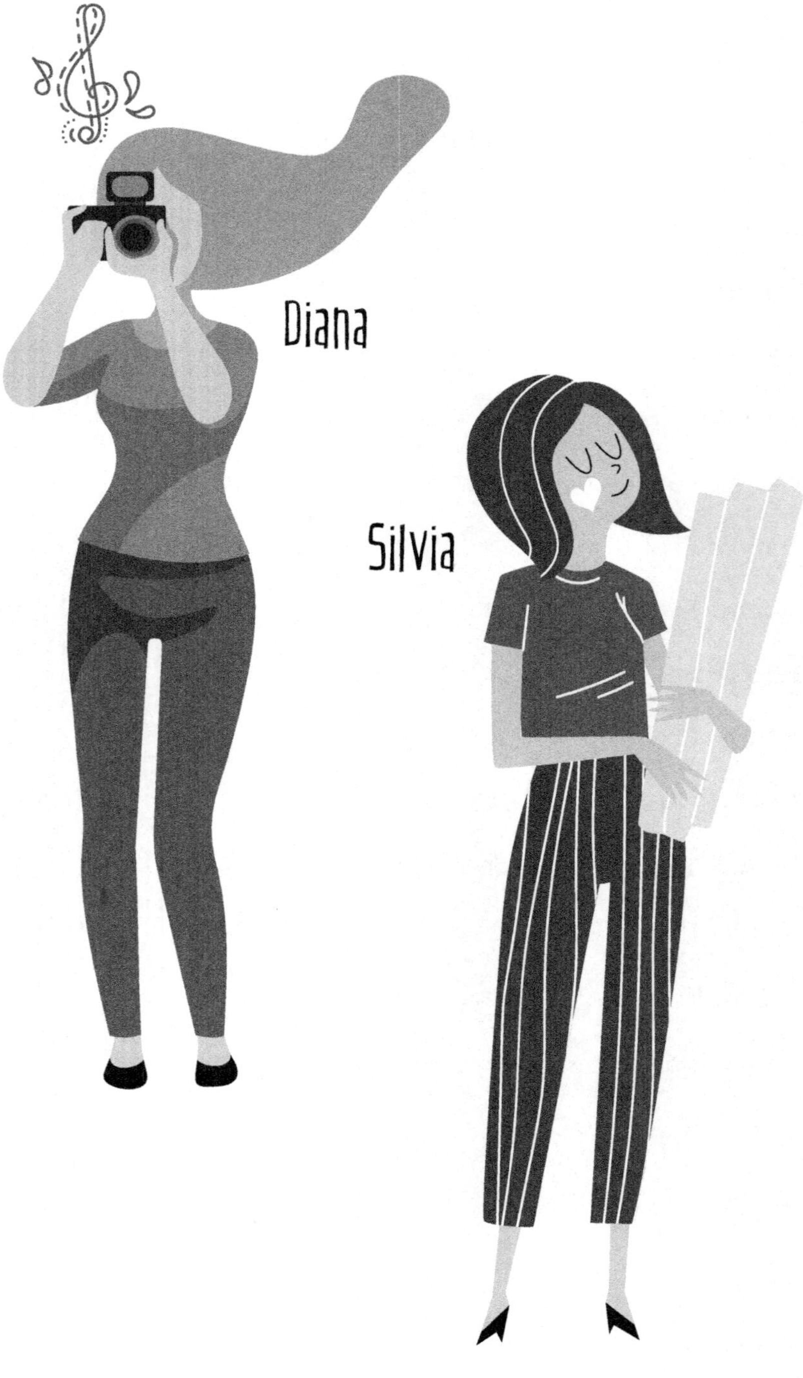
Diana
Silvia

INTRODUCTION

A Simple and Effective Diet

Are you struggling to lose weight or wanting to shift that stubborn fat from your tummy or hips? Do you hate diets with all the restriction on the delicious foods you love? Well, I may just have a solution that could help.

Let me introduce myself. I'm Diana, originally from Argentina but now based in the coastal city of Brighton, UK, where I've lived for over three decades. I'm also a mother of three children and a grandmother of one, and at five-feet-eight, I'm a toned size 10 and weigh only nine and a half stones (approx. 60 kilos).

Friends often say I am living proof that you can enjoy a variety of so-called 'naughty' foods such as pizza, spaghetti, chocolate cake, doughnuts or even a glass of wine and still stay slim and healthy.

That's easy for you to say, you might think, you must have a fast metabolism. Well, the truth is, my slender figure has nothing to do with a fast metabolism or lucky genetics. I simply embarked on a unique way of eating that had nothing to do with what you eat and everything to do with when you eat? And it's something that can be achieved by anyone. Let me explain.

Over twenty years ago, I was a student of 80-year-old French dietary pioneer, Pierre Marion. Young in spirit, Pierre's reputation preceded him and people travelled from all corners of the globe to his office in Hove on the south coast of England to lose weight and be treated for many types of illness such as rheumatoid arthritis, spondylitis, sciatica, irritable bowel syndrome, severe acne and psoriasis. Indeed, many ailments that doctors couldn't help with were cured by his unique dietary techniques. His success rate was phenomenal and spread through word of mouth along with his successful book, *Eat and Be Happy* (now out of print).

My former-husband, Glen, had a lung condition that couldn't be diagnosed, and was constantly coughing and struggling to breathe. Within three months, these issues were resolved through this dietary eating plan. Anyone Pierre agreed to treat, however, had to first follow his dynamic digestive regime for a period of time, a method which enabled the human body to replenish and heal itself to such an extent that further treatment was often rendered unnecessary, and along with this healing, the patient's body weight was also significantly reduced. Not only this – the excess fat was reduced only in the places where it accumulated – around the midriff, the upper arms and buttocks, for example, restoring the body to its natural shape.

Pierre would often show bewildered amusement at the way some of his patients placed weight loss as one of the great benefits of his treatment. To him, restoration of health was the paramount concern, and then, when digestion was back in balance, a slimmer body shape was the result.

Silvia, my co-author who lives in Madrid working as a successful architect, in her early fifties, had developed an eye condition called macular degeneration which causes severe vision loss. Over two months of following Pierre's strict regime of eating meals before 9 a.m., she was able to see clearly. As an additional benefit, she'd slimmed down from a size sixteen to a size twelve. She complained that her clothes were now far too loose and she'd have to get them taken in – that had not been part of the plan, but needless to say, she was very happy about the result!

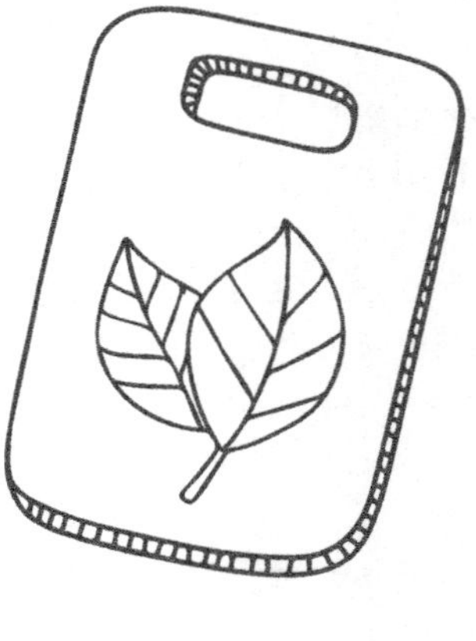

As his student, however, I found his approach to eating my main meal before nine in the morning extremely difficult to maintain with any kind of busy lifestyle and over the last ten years, Silvia and I have adapted his method around working hours, social, and family life to come up with a new system - one which is as successful at achieving sustainable weight loss and improving health as the much stricter dietary rules which underpinned the original methodology.

Hence the title 'Before 2' – and it's exactly that – you eat what you want before two in the afternoon. This approach to eating can lead to wonderful results – not just in terms of weight loss but a noticeable improvement in muscle and skin tone, physique and general health. And the secret is this: it's not a matter of what you eat, it's the time of day that you eat your food which is crucial.

Now, I don't claim to be giving you a heal-all for myriad health disorders in the way that Pierre was able to – but as you read this book, you'll see how this regime, simple as it is, can bring exhilarating, life-changing results. Your eyes will sparkle as the blood flow to your skin is replenished, muscles regain their tautness, flexibility is restored, and you'll lose that cumbersome excess weight.

Diets can offer weight loss, but few result in diminishing the accumulation of body fat that won't shift from stubborn places such as the thighs, hips or tummy. As Pierre would say in his strong French accent, quoting an English proverb that delighted him enormously, "The proof of the pudding is in the eating." Or as I say, try it – you'll like it!

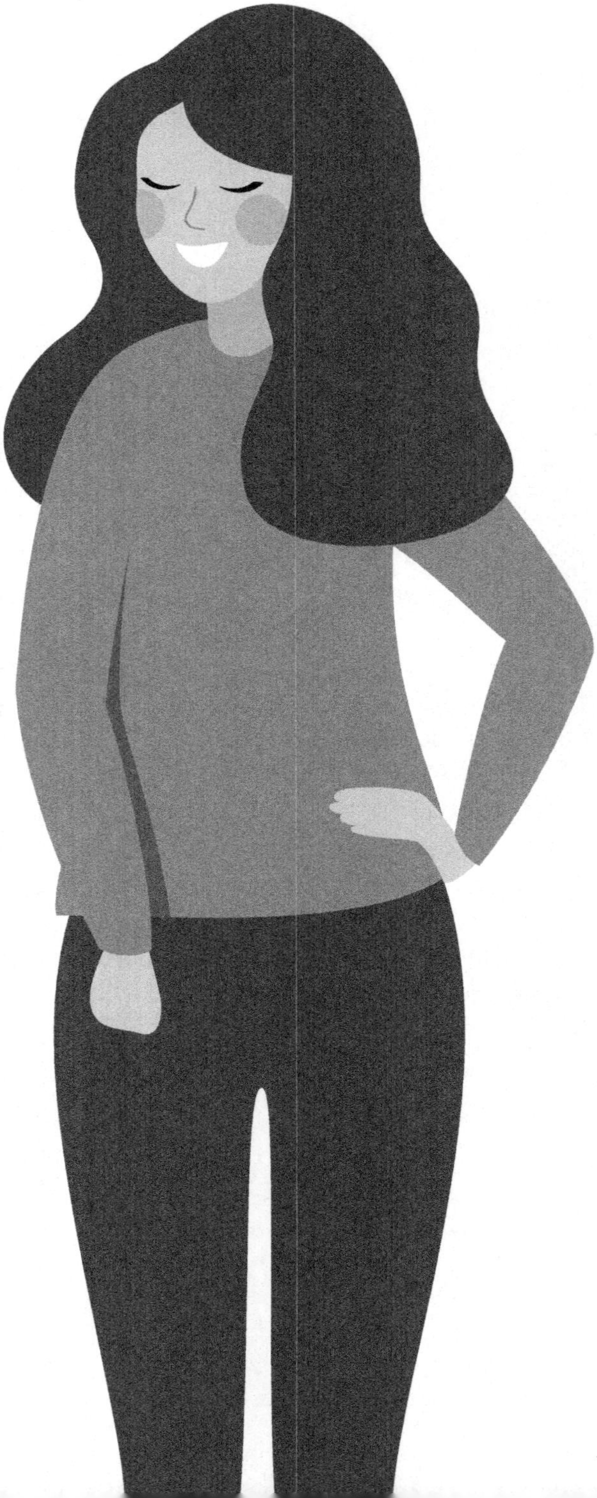

chapter one

Breakfast Like a King

CHAPTER ONE

Breakfast Like a King

In the days of old, it was taken as read that one should breakfast like a king, lunch like a courtier, and sup like a pauper. We can see from well-researched television documentaries and books how the inhabitants of medieval life such as farmers, craftsmen and masons with their backbreaking labour needed the stamina and strength provided by a hearty breakfast to get through the day.

Today's modern world is a complete contrast. We stuff ourselves with snacks throughout the day, almost habitually, not because we're hungry but simply because we fancy that bag of crisps or a bar of chocolate, and naturally, it's normal isn't it, to dunk a few cookies into our cup of coffee or tea every time we have one. And then we go on to eat a heavy meal in the evening, giving the contents of our stomach no chance to be properly digested before we finally collapse into sleep. And worse still, placing our bodies in a horizontal position in bed is the worst thing for our digestion, because the food in our stomach lays there sluggishly until morning, turning slowly into body fat.

Is it any wonder that obesity is the scourge of modern society? It's all around us and proliferating at an alarming rate where overweight children, teens and adults are commonplace. Back in the early 1940s when rationing during WWII was part of everyday life, obesity was rare, because people couldn't sate their desires whenever they felt like it – there were boundaries in place to stop you.

So, we need to take some tips from the past and learn how our ancestors from the middle ages instinctively got their eating routines right, because the essential secret of 'Before 2' is to wake up famished and eat ravenously. Whether your lifestyle means you're desk-bound or active, everything is about the digestion of food in the early part of the day, where you can enjoy the biggest of breakfasts and a feast for lunch.

As we all know, protein and carbohydrates are needed for our body, though you might wonder, aren't we supposed to avoid carbs? Well, no, actually... we're not. The fact is that pasta, bread, cakes, and potatoes can be enjoyed too, without any guilt.

Following this Before 2 regime, you won't need to count calories, weigh out portion-controlled food or buy those watery soups and flavourless milkshakes. The key lies in the time you eat your meal. If you've finally finished a large portion of spaghetti carbonara along with every last crumb of chocolate cake and double cream before 2 p.m., you will still lose weight easily. And you'll notice how fit and energised you'll feel too.

Fasting from Two O'Clock

2 p.m. is the cut-off point. After this, you cannot eat any food – zilch, zero, nada – until your breakfast the next morning. It sounds challenging but after a week or two, you'll get used to it.

Drink as much as you like, though, as long as your beverage isn't considered a food – so that means, nothing with milk or pulp – no cups of milky tea, lattes, smoothies or milkshakes. Instead, you can have a cup of herbal tea, a black tea or coffee, non-pulpy fruit juice or even a glass of wine.

But the zero food intake means that by the time you retire, whether it's around ten o'clock or midnight, your body will have finished digesting all the contents from earlier in the day, and you'll be going to bed on an empty stomach. This is essential as will soon become clear.

To Eat or Not to Eat, That is the Question

Many people have a distinct dislike of diets and understandably so. Most of the time they don't work as when we stop them, the pounds pile up again in double quick time. Despite this, there's a wide selection of diet books in the bookstore – clear proof that trying to lose weight has become one of the greatest social obsessions of the modern age.

Dieting is all about reducing your intake of certain foods. In particular, they advise us to avoid at all costs the very foods we enjoy the most. So, is there a malevolent god somewhere who's playing with us, offering us the most delicious delicacies and treats, that we must then deny in the interests of looking slim?

Our advice is to do just the opposite. You can enjoy the food you like. Eat until you're fit to burst – simply do it early in the day and before the cut-off time of 2 p.m. This is the most powerful secret in the science of weight loss.

It sounds ridiculous, doesn't it? It goes against every possible instinct of the dieting process. But with this method, your main meal at breakfast or lunchtime can be – if you desire – a slap-up three or four-course feast of gourmet proportions. You can then use your free time in the late afternoon or early evening for sport, a yoga class, studying, catching up on Netflix or simply reading your latest novel.

In simple terms, as you read on, you'll receive insight into your body and its digestive functioning that will help you understand how this eating method can give you the healthy weight and trim physique that you truly deserve.

chapter two

Getting Started

CHAPTER TWO

Getting Started

'Before 2' is a digestive regime which cleans out the body, enhances your appearance and leads to impressive weight reduction. And the great secret is simply this: it's not a matter of what you eat, it's the time of day that you eat that's crucial.

- We know that a new weight-loss plan can be overwhelming especially if you're used to eating a big evening meal. The best way to prepare for this new way of eating is to make gradual changes – eat less at night and more in the morning until you feel ready to cut out your evening meal altogether. If you've not been to the doctors for a while, it wouldn't be a bad idea to have a check-up to find out your general health condition such as blood pressure, cholesterol, and so on...

- When you're ready to stop eating at 2 p.m., you can start, this will allow you to feel the full benefits of this diet immediately. After just a few days, you'll notice that you've begun to feel lighter and healthier. If you've cheated one evening and devoured that large bag of nachos, don't give up, just get back into your stride the next day with a big breakfast, brunch or lunch.

- Take your body measurements – the scales don't always tell you the full story – so measure yourself around your chest, waist and hips. Write the measurements down in inches on a notepad and put it away somewhere safe. But update your measurements and weigh yourself only once a fortnight, otherwise, it can easily become an obsession. Congratulations – you are **ON YOUR WAY!**

- Go to bed on an empty stomach. You won't have eaten since two o'clock that day and you will wake up ravenously hungry. Maybe get up one hour before you start your day, so you can prepare and enjoy your meal without stress, or prepare a meal the night before that you can simply heat up.

With a big meal, say three courses with a main meal, salad and a dessert, you need to drink at least two litres of liquid. So, remember to prepare plenty to drink: a teapot full of your choice of tea, a jug of water or fruit juice. When you get used to enjoying this morning or lunchtime meal, it's helpful to your digestion if you can develop the habit of taking a drink every two spoonfuls of food. Drinking a lot of liquid with your food is very important as will become clear in later chapters.

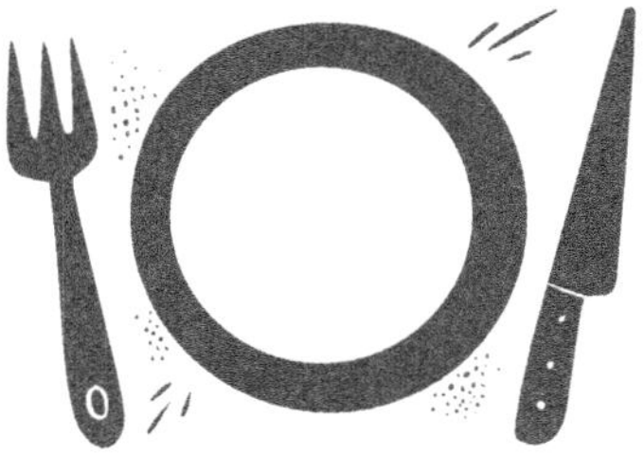

Your meal should be nutritious, comprising of protein and carbs with freshly prepared vegetables. This will be the main meal of your day, so enjoy something sweet afterwards - a dessert or a piece of cake as long as you finish before 2 p.m.

FYI A FAST TRACK for losing weight

To recap, the hours when you can eat are between 5 a.m. and 2 p.m.

If you need to lose weight faster, the earlier in the day you finish eating, the quicker you'll lose weight.

The later you eat in the day, the slower you'll lose weight.

If you wish, you can stay on this diet forever; you'll never be underweight. Your body will reach whatever weight and shape it naturally needs to remain healthy.

The good news is that this diet works whether you're overweight or underweight. If you're overweight, you'll lose kilos and inches, and if you're underweight, you'll fill out in all the right places. It sounds incredible but it's true. Either way, you'll achieve the best body shape for you.

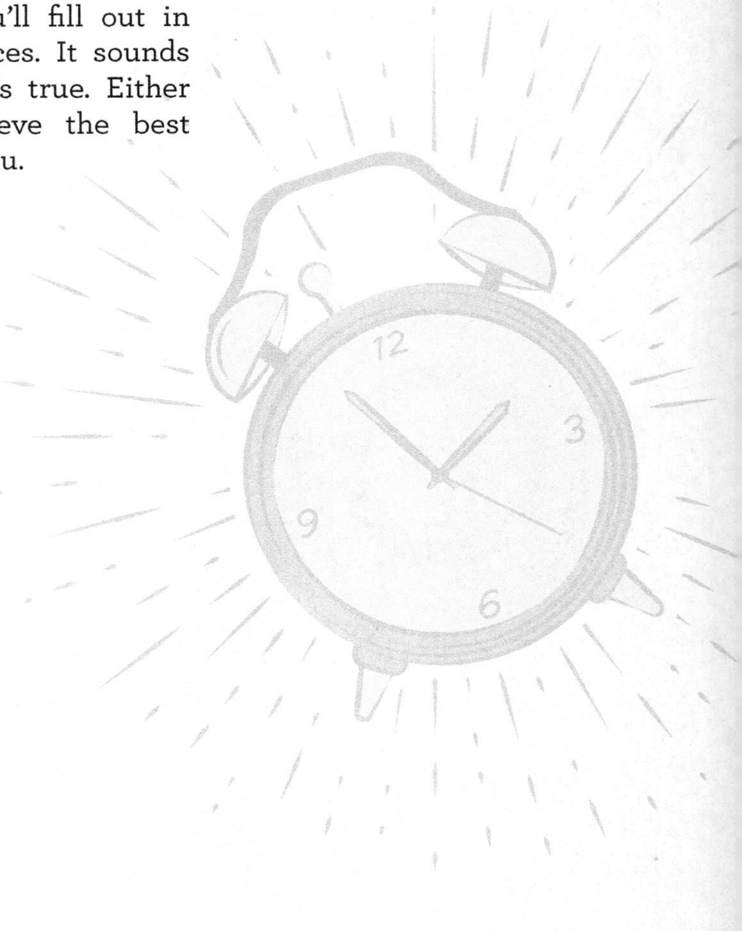

chapter three

The Fast

CHAPTER THREE

The Fast

After 2 p.m., no food must pass your lips until you wake up the following morning.

You can drink anything you like, but it must be without milk, without pulp, and without salt or sugar unless it's cane sugar. All other sugars, for example, corn syrup or artificial sweeteners will start your digestion process working again as they need to be digested – so stick to only black coffee, black tea, herb tea or water without sugar unless you can guarantee it's cane sugar. But we don't recommend too much coffee after 2 p.m. as it might affect your sleep.

If you feel famished before bedtime, a few glasses of water or herbal tea will fill you up and you'll know that, when you wake up, you can have an enjoyable big breakfast.

You could have a hot drink with honey, too. Honey is interesting dietary-wise. If you eat it straight from the jar, it has to be digested, but if it's diluted in a hot drink, it's not activating the digestive process.

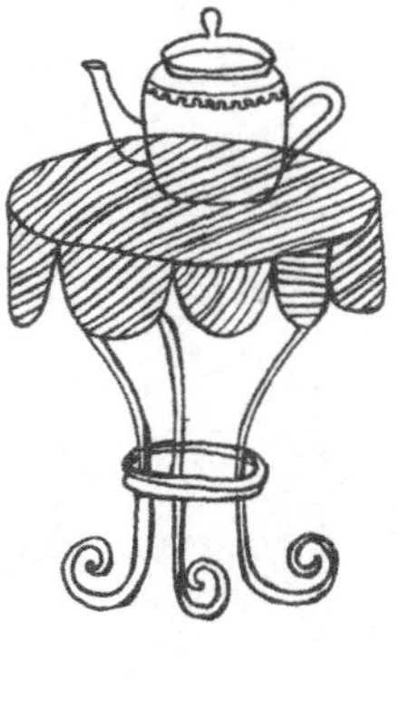

Intermittent fasting is one of the biggest trends today and the science behind it reveals many of its health benefits – but the only time fasting is really useful is during the night while we're asleep. This can only happen if we don't eat from 2 p.m.

Neuroscientist, Dr Matthew Walker, said: "If I measure your brainwave activity with electrodes, I can see a drop in your physiological alertness between 2 p.m. and 4 p.m. when it's genetically hard-wired to drop." It's at this time of the day when the activity of the digestive system slows down and later in the day stops altogether.

If we tried fasting in the morning it would also disrupt our circadian rhythms – the time our body clocks are set up for the activity of feeding the body. (More on circadian rhythms in the next chapter). In addition, the importance of fasting from 2 p.m. is to sleep on an empty stomach, so that the digestive system is at rest during these hours. This enables the body to strengthen the immune system, eliminate toxins, renew cells, and burn fat.

People assume that if we feel hungry later on in the day, it's because we're starving and need to eat. This is far from the truth when we've already had one or two big meals before 2 p.m. And this early meal should be a real feast to keep you going well into the evening. So, if you feel hungry, it could be because you've not had enough food earlier in the day.

The liver is the organ which stabilises glucose. One of the liver's main tasks is to maintain glucose circulating through the blood; it stores and manufactures glucose depending upon the body's need. When we eat sugar or carbohydrates, the body releases glucose into the bloodstream immediately, triggering the production of insulin. When the levels of insulin are high, the body links chains of glucose together into a compound called glycogen which is then stored in the liver for the time when we're not eating. When levels drop, the liver turns glycogen back into glucose and releases it into the bloodstream. This important role of the liver will work more efficiently when we don't eat late in the afternoon and evening.

The bile in the liver also picks up the waste and moves it into the intestines. In addition the kidneys will filter the blood passing waste out of the body through the urine. Only when we stop eating at 2 p.m. does the body maximise the detoxifying and cleaning processes of the food we've eaten. After a few days on this diet, you'll wake up in the morning feeling the difference a clean digestive system has made.

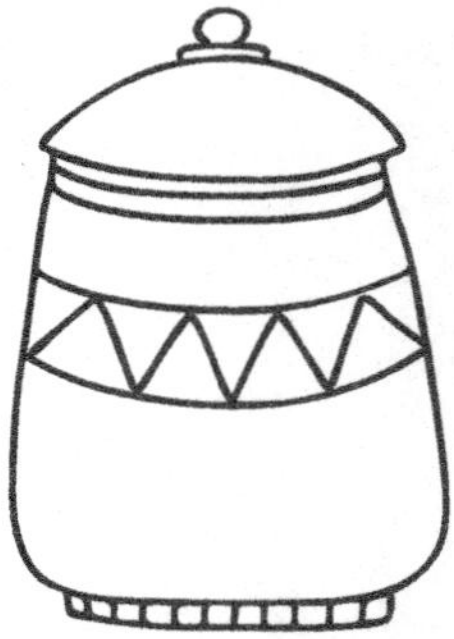

How to deal with a night out on the Before 2 diet

It's fair to say that this eating regime can present restrictions to your social life as people often get together for dinner or drinks in the evening. On the odd occasion, you can break this fast to eat with friends, but if it's a regular social night out and you want to maintain our eating plan for long term benefits, then organise meeting your friends for lunch or for evening drinks instead. Because, remember, you can still enjoy the odd glass of wine, beer or vodka, which won't affect your fast as long as it's not got salt or pulp in it. So, no Bloody Marys, Piña Coladas or Tequilas.

We can then feel content that we're treating ourselves to the best of both worlds. And don't be surprised if after a couple of weeks those friends embracing this method will assess your slimmer, healthier physique and ask: "Will it work for me as it's obviously working for you?"

So, remember that any extra food consumed later in the day won't get used as fuel and will instead be stored as fat within the body which can lead to weight gain. After two weeks, you should no longer feel hungry in the evening as your body acclimatises to this new routine.

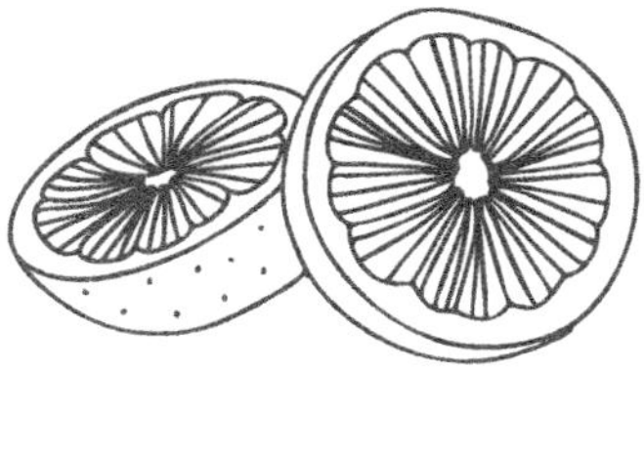

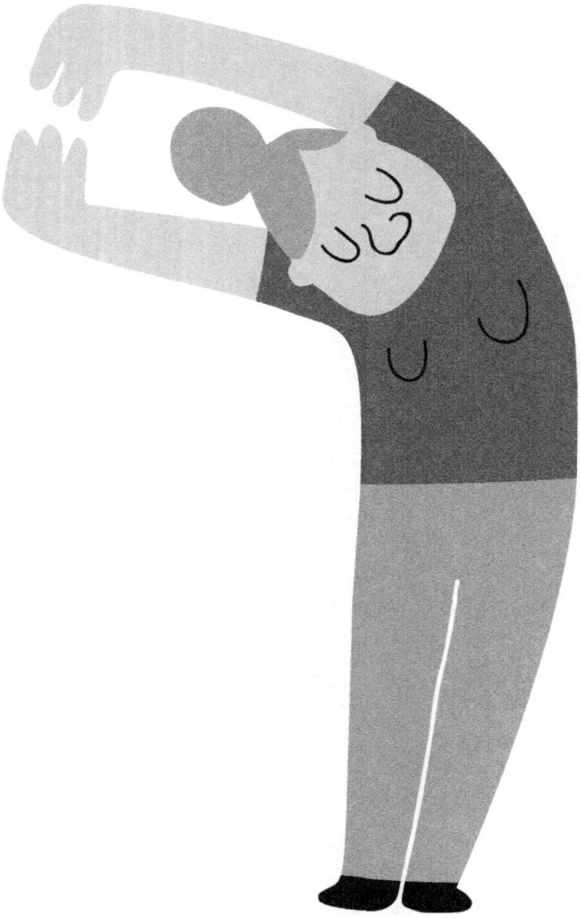

chapter four

Body Clocks and Rhythms

CHAPTER FOUR

Body Clocks and Rhythms

A biological study has caused quite a stir since it first appeared in the 1990s – the circadian rhythms, the study of changes in our bodies over 24 hours. So, what are the circadian rhythms and why are they important?
In simple terms, they represent the influence of the sun in every aspect of life on this planet. People, plants and animals have these built-in cycles which allow them to eat and sleep at the right time. These rhythms consist of internal clocks which are re-set by time signals such as sunrise and sunset. As you may notice, there are certain times during the day when you'll feel more alert than others. These rhythms regulate many bodily functions including eating, sleeping, body temperature and hormone production.

A simple way to identify the effects of circadian rhythms is by travelling across time zones and experiencing for oneself the unpleasant effects of jet lag. The distress associated with jet lag is felt when our circadian rhythms become out of sync with the new time zone. Therefore, losing or gaining time during air travel can leave us feeling disoriented, especially if our bodies expect daylight when it's actually dark or vice versa. Eventually, the body adjusts its body clocks to the new environment, and wellbeing can resume.

These rhythms are controlled by a master clock in the brain which resets every day with the rising of the sun. Like the cockerel's song at the crack of dawn, ready to get a head start on his daily hunt for food, his master body clock is telling him that it's time wake up and eat.

When the sun goes down, the master clock in our brain sends a signal to the pituitary gland to release a hormone called melatonin which makes us feel tired. For many, this tiredness occurs around seven or eight in the evening. You might also notice a regular time when you become sleepy.

These clocks and rhythms are so inherent we hardly notice them, but they influence everything going on in our physical systems throughout the day and night. In fact, every organ in the body has its own internal clock.

Our master clock is located at the base of the brain, called the hypothalamus in the suprachiasmatic nucleus which detects the light coming through our pupils. For example, researchers from the Harvard Medical School have now discovered a light sensor at the back of the eye, totally separate from our vision sensors, which observes the changes in light throughout the day and passes this information to the master clock in our brain and then sends a signal to the other body clocks which adjust accordingly.

Our body clocks are groups of cells which tell all parts of the body what time it is and what needs to be done. These changes mean there are optimum times of the day for certain activities. As a result, the complex processes at work in the digestion of food have come under scrutiny – thus discovering the optimum time to eat and digest food has given us an entirely new understanding in intelligent eating, good health, and weight loss.

Before 2 follows these natural rhythms of the body. This means any type of food we eat early in the day – when the brain sends a signal to the body that it's time to eat – will be turned into energy. And any toxins will also be expelled from our body.

When we don't eat at the correct hour, our body clocks reset themselves as they are then out of sync and this can cause health problems such as obesity and premature ageing.

Professors Marta Garaulet and Jose M. Ordovas, authors of *Chronobiology and Obesity,* have conducted experiments on how circadian rhythms relate to food consumption. Their findings show that the digestive system's efficiency levels are very sensitive to the time of day and reach their peak at around 8 a.m. an optimum time to have eaten food. The work of their team has shed light on the importance of timing in the digestive process.

Researchers from Brigham and Women's Hospital in Massachusetts have also produced research on this subject, collaborating with the University of Murcia in Spain and Tufts University in Massachusetts. They found that it's not simply what you eat, but also what time you eat, that may help with weight loss.

Their study was published in 2013 in the *International Journal of Obesity.* The researchers studied 420 overweight participants who followed a 20 week weight-loss programme. They formed two groups, one eating their main meal before 3 p.m. and the other eating their main meal after 3 p.m. It was found that the early-eaters lost significantly more weight than the late-eaters.

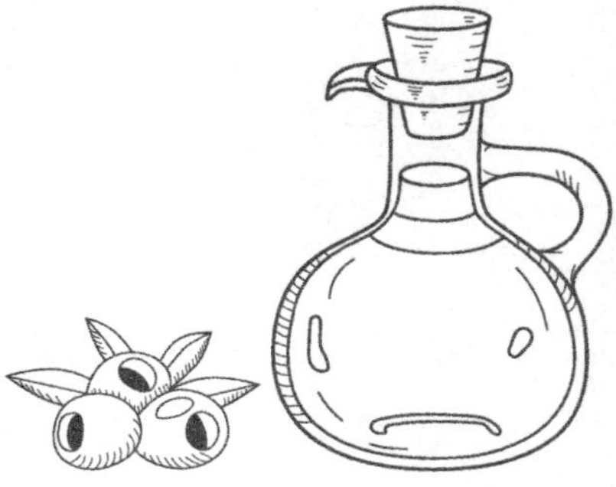

This research reveals how the process of digestion is dependent on the time of day, and how the food we eat will be turned into energy when eaten earlier. Pierre Marion discovered that the best time to eat was before 9 a.m. as revealed by Professors Garaulet and Ordovas. However, we discovered this was socially impossible to fit around work and family life for most people, which is why we reframed his programme into a new concept: 'Before 2'.

What we've noticed is that at 2 p.m. there's a dip in the energy of the digestive system and anything we eat after 2 p.m. will float around in the stomach for hours, adversely affecting our energy and concentration. Digestion itself will take up to a third of your body's energy. So although we say Before 2, the earlier you eat in the day, the better.

The logic and insight of the digestive process we also say, make a powerful case for trying Before 2. It's simple and straightforward.

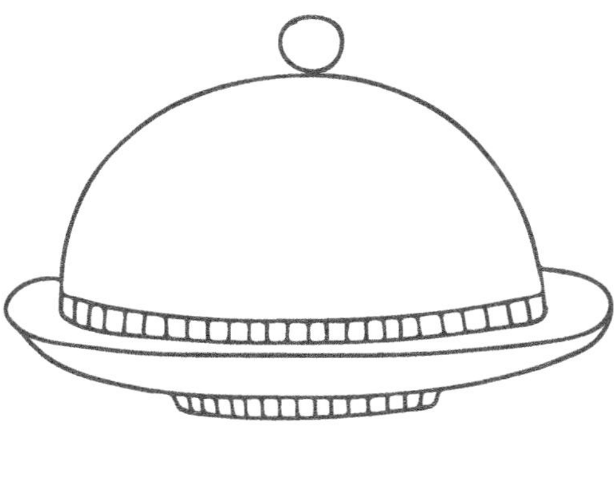

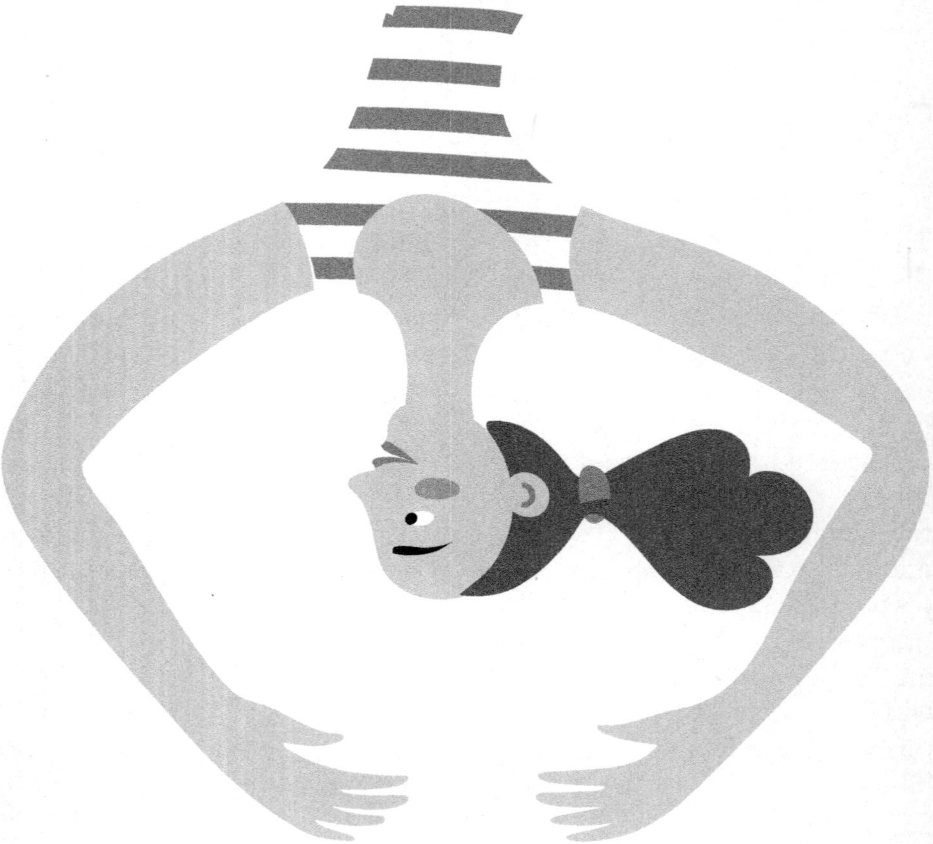

chapter five

Gravity at Work

CHAPTER FIVE

Gravity at Work

When gravity was discovered, it explained a lot of scientific mysteries. For example, why we stand on the earth instead of falling off it, why the earth orbits the sun, and explains the movement of the tides. Gravity is everywhere, we hardly give it a second thought. But gravity also plays an important part in our digestion.

When we eat, food is chewed, swallowed and moved through the oesophagus where waves of contractions transport it into the stomach. The muscles in the stomach then help to mix and break down the food by churning it around in gastric acid. Gravity then plays a major role, representing the only way food can travel into the small intestine – because only when we're upright, standing or sitting, can food pass through the stomach towards our intestine. If we're lying down, without the pull of gravity, the stomach cannot empty itself, despite the efforts made by the muscular contractions. Digestion will simply stop. And because of the position of the stomach when we lie down, there's also a risk of heartburn caused by acid reflux as it flows back into the oesophagus.

If you live in a country where a siesta is a routine, we'd recommend that you don't lie down after 2 p.m. as this will hinder the digestive process. Alternatively, you could have a snooze in an armchair ensuring your torso remains upright so food can continue to pass through to the lower intestine.

Therein lies the problem if you eat a meal in the evening – the food remains in the stomach all night long to fester. Why is that a problem? Think about it... if you leave warm food out overnight, bacteria will form by morning, because the food has begun to putrefy. That's what happens when you leave food to stew overnight in your stomach's gastric acid. Putrefaction begins – not enough to cause immediate illness, but over time it creates toxins in the body that lead to lethargy and ill-health.

But most importantly – when the body doesn't have to work on digesting the contents of your gut overnight, it can revert to its normal functions: resting, repairing and renewing cells, and burning up excess fat. That's why it's so important to go to bed on an empty stomach.

This all sounds very technical, but all you need to know is: ensure you don't lie down after eating your meal and go to bed on an empty stomach. That's because an average meal can take anything from four to seven hours to digest, and why it's better not to eat any food after 2 p.m.

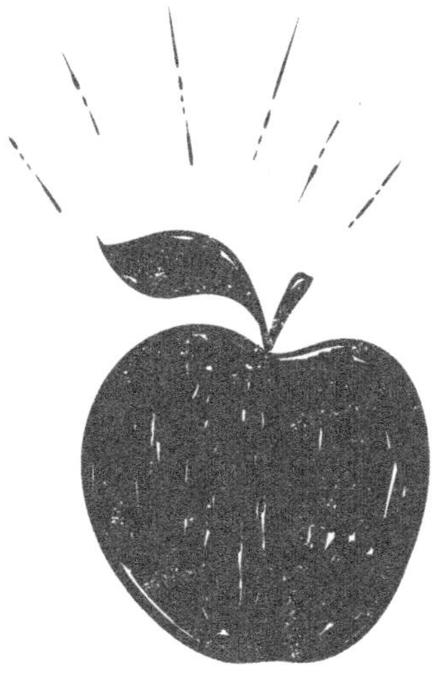

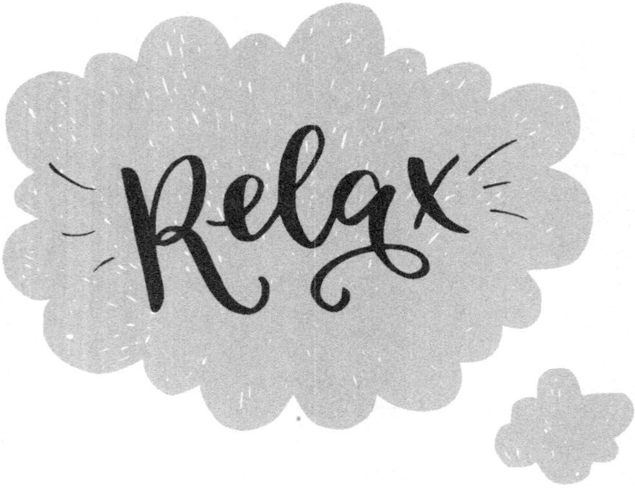
Relax

chapter six

Beauty Sleep

CHAPTER SIX

Beauty Sleep

With our new lifestyle eating regime, you're heading to bed on an empty stomach – so, let's not put too fine a point on it, you may be a little hungry, especially if you've skipped the midday meal or haven't eaten enough, and especially during the early stages of your progress. We'd advise you to be prepared – don't be tempted to open the fridge door whilst you're watching a movie on Netflix and looking for something to snack on. Don't do it! Put that chocolate bar down. No munchies!

We can fight these cravings by developing an early to bed regime. This means that when you wake up early to prepare the meal you've been dreaming about, you're going to be wide awake. Alternatively, if it's hard to get an early night because of work, you can prepare a meal the night before and store it in the fridge, ready to be warmed up the next day.

As mentioned in the previous chapter, lying down halts the force of gravity so the body can rest, heal, and restore cells, burn fat, and fight off any harmful viruses.

Getting good quality sleep is one of the best things we can do for weight loss and our health. Sleep is also important for our brain, a process called memory consolidation, where the brain processes feelings and memories from our day, eliminating the ones we don't need, a bit like scanning and cleaning your computer.

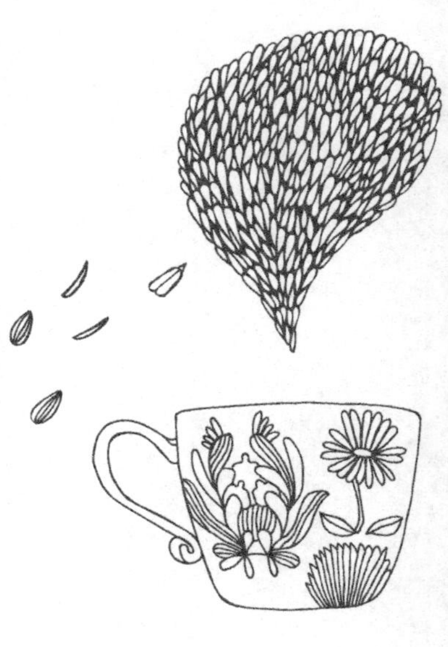

The loss of daylight informs our master clock that night is now in session, so the body releases melatonin which is a signal to our brain and body that it's time for bed. For this reason, it's important to sleep in a room with thick curtains. Any light seeping into the room during sleep suppresses melatonin production which controls sleep and wake cycles as well as the growth hormone which is essential for tissue repair. Another hormone, cortisol, takes a dip at bedtime and starts peaking just before we wake up. This hormone is a wake-up signal to our body, that switches on our energy and our appetite.

Checking emails, online shopping, texting or checking social media an hour before bed is also not advised. It may seem harmless enough, but the sleep disruption caused by these blue light-emitting devices is significantly higher and more harmful than an electric light. Instead, replace the habit with a good book or a magazine.

Those who are used to going to bed late, say after midnight, could try going to bed half an hour earlier. If you don't feel tired at least lie down so the body is in a restful position, and then gradually get into bed a little earlier every night.

We all wish we could get by on less sleep, but it's such an important part of our lives. However, it's not just the amount of hours we sleep that counts, it's the quality that's important. There's an assumption that a nap taken during the day can repair the lack of a good night's sleep, but this isn't the case. The sleep between 8 p.m. and 6 a.m. is the best quality sleep you can have. And when sleeping on an empty stomach, the body can do an even deeper cellular repair and burn fat whereas, when your stomach is full, the body is investing a lot of energy simply trying to digest food.

That's why we recommend early to bed, whenever you can. As neuroscientist Matthew Walker says in his book *Why We Sleep:* "It's time for us to reclaim our right to a full night of sleep without embarrassment or the damaging stigma of laziness."

Naturally, the sleep requirement varies with each person, but we recommend around eight hours, although some may need more. In general, people who go to bed early need less sleep than those who go to bed later. When we get less sleep than our body needs, as well as affecting memory and performance, it weakens our health.

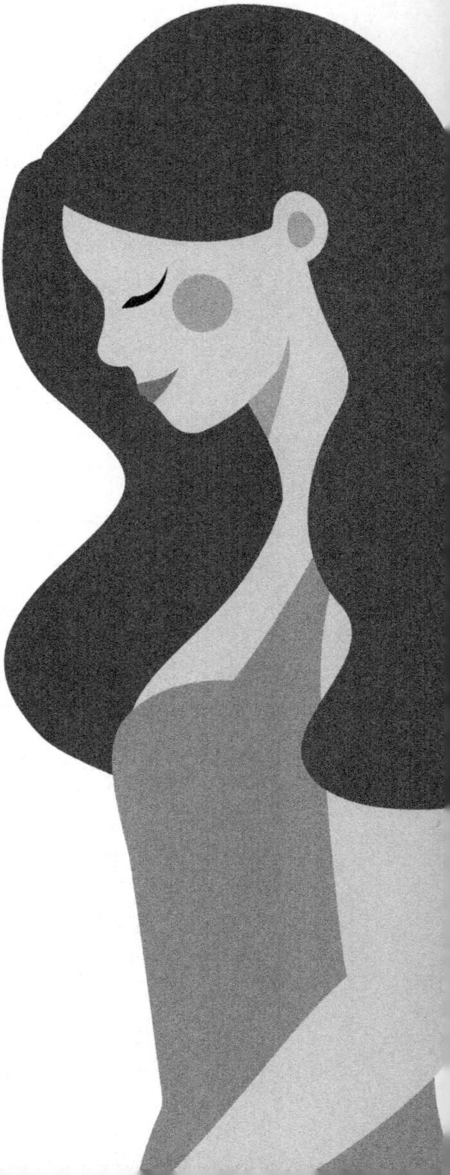

chapter seven

To Drink or Not to Drink

CHAPTER SEVEN

To Drink or not to Drink

You may be surprised to hear that drinking plenty of liquid during meals helps digestion a great deal. Drinking helps soften food and move it down the oesophagus towards the stomach. When the food reaches the stomach, the gastric juices produced there are in direct relation to the volume of liquid taken with a meal – the more liquid is mixed with the food, the more gastric juices will be produced, contrary to the persistent myth that we shouldn't drink with our meal. In fact, there's no scientific evidence that drinking during a meal could negatively affect the digestion or absorption of nutrients.

To clarify, the main function of the digestive system is to break food down into small molecules to be used for energy, growth, and cellular repair. The digestive process starts in the mouth where saliva glands and any liquids we drink moisten our food, so that it slides more easily into the stomach. After food and drink enter the stomach, they mix with the digestive juices and hydrochloric acid – a process which continues as the stomach slowly empties its contents into the small intestine where nutrients are absorbed into your bloodstream. The waste products then shift into the large intestine.

Unlike our ancestors, the apes, we have developed a longer small intestine and a shorter large intestine, creating a much more advanced digestive system, better for absorbing a wider variety of food, giving us the nutrients to develop a more advanced brain and nervous system.

We cannot emphasise how important it is for the body to stay hydrated. We can survive around three weeks without food, but can only survive three days without water. The blood in our body is made up of 90% water, our brain is 85% water, and the rest of our body is around 60% water.

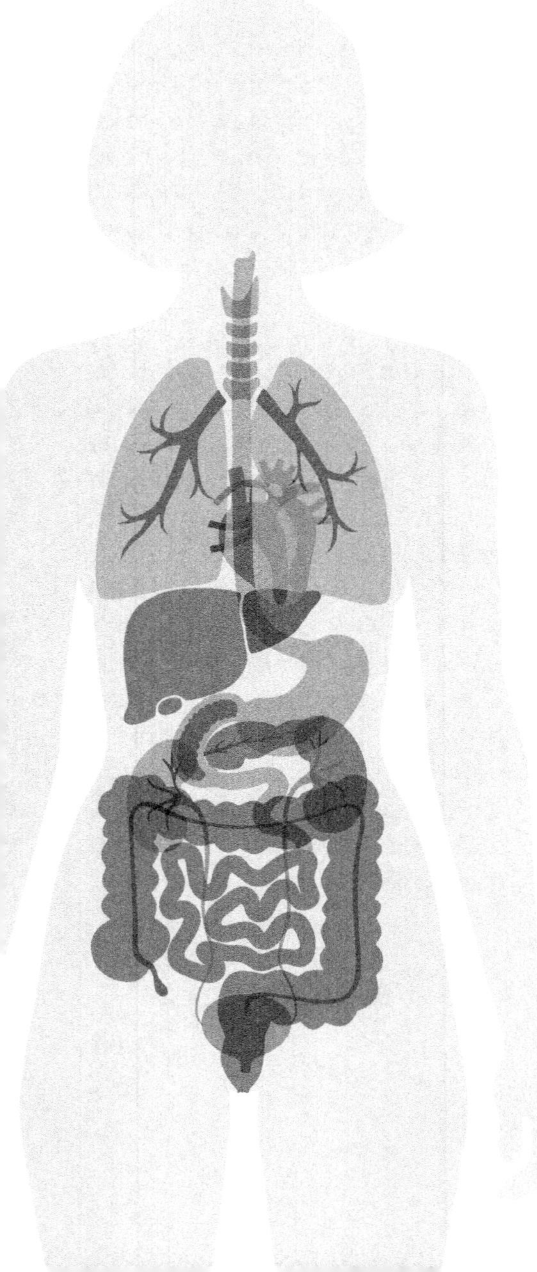

If we don't drink enough with our meal, the food in our stomach won't have sufficient gastric juices for digestion which enables bacteria to grow, and we could then suffer from indigestion.

To explain further, when food passes from the stomach into the intestines, it becomes a fluid called 'chyle'. The milkier this substance is, the more it's able to feed the blood with nutrients. Without liquid, the food we eat becomes a sticky paste which makes the digestive process more challenging. The undigested food then ferments in the small intestine, feeding bacteria and the hydrochloric acid cannot penetrate through the layers of food to kill all the bacteria.

So, although it's necessary to drink throughout the day, the optimum time to drink liquid is during meals. Drinking after a meal won't have the same significant effect on digestion as it's too late for the liquid to produce gastric juices to break down the contents.

The time your food remains in the stomach depends on the consistency of what you've eaten and the amount of liquid taken with the food. It also depends on the time of day that you eat. An evening meal will digest fifty per cent slower than the same meal taken during the morning hours. But if food is properly chewed and plenty of fluid is drunk during the meal, the digestion will not only be faster, but the stomach acid will kill most of the bacteria and enable an enzyme called pepsin to work more efficiently, breaking down the nutrients and eliminating the food the body doesn't need.

In summary, if we don't digest our food fully, the body simply doesn't produce the nutrients needed for optimum health.

Of course, it needn't be just a glass of water with a meal, it could also be fruit juice or tea or coffee, but for optimum benefits, it's best to drink at least two litres of liquid during a three-course meal, and more, if you want to.

Although we must point out that we're not talking about alcoholic drinks as alcohol has the opposite effect, causing the body to dehydrate. The nutrients need to end up 'shaped' into a form that can be absorbed into the bloodstream. This process is the job of the digestive enzymes. Enzymes require a high level of water in their structures to deliver their full functionality, which is why drinking a lot with our meals is an essential component of the Before 2 diet.

When we eat our meal, we should chew each mouthful completely before taking the next bite and take a drink every two mouthfuls.

Warm drinks help our digestion more than chilled drinks – our body temperature is 37°C and anything we eat or drink should ideally be equal to this temperature. If what we drink is lower, it will slow down the emptying of the stomach.

So, enjoy your meal with plenty of liquids, select good quality food, and prepare it so that it looks and tastes delicious. We also recommend that you take some time away from your busy schedule to give you time to properly enjoy the pleasure of eating, even if you're sitting at the dining table alone.

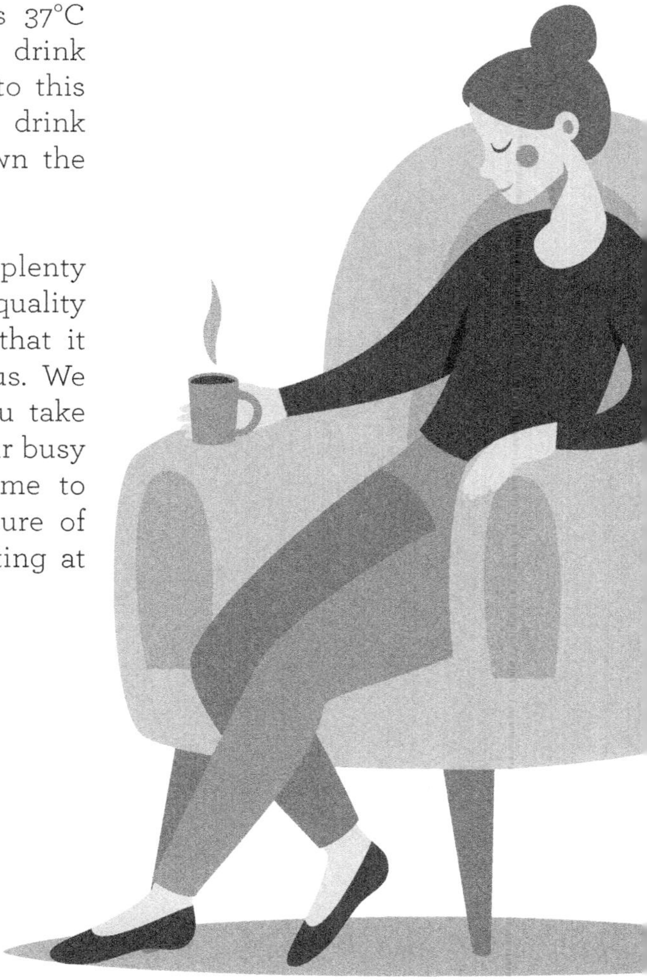

chapter eight

Sugar is not Sugar

CHAPTER EIGHT

Sugar is not Sugar

The food we call sugar gives our body energy. It comes from a carbohydrate called sucrose which in turn is made of fructose and glucose. The word glucose comes from the Greek word for 'sweet'. Apart from adding a sweet flavour to our food, it's essential to our body – our brains use up to four hundred calories of glucose every day. If the glucose in our blood is low, we feel tired. We may also feel the signs of stress, anxiety and irritability.

Nature is wise and provides all the nutrition needed for our body. For example, human breast milk is noticeably sweeter than cow's milk and there's a good reason for that. It contains a lot of glucose which a baby needs to feed the brain. Most of us love sugar, although some crave it more than others, sugar makes up the backbone of our DNA. It helps power our cells and store energy for later – and it doesn't make us fat. In fact, it's a basic biological need. Our body is designed to keep the level of glucose in the blood constant. Most of the cells in our body use glucose, and glucose is also the main source of fuel for our brain. But sugar is sugar, right? Actually, no – there are many different types of sugar – some are good, and others are bad for our health.

Sugar comes from the sugarcane plant or sugar beet. Both of them are 99.95% sucrose, even though they come from different plants. These are the good sugars and the most efficient source of energy for our body as they don't need to be digested, passing quickly through the walls of the small intestine into the bloodstream.

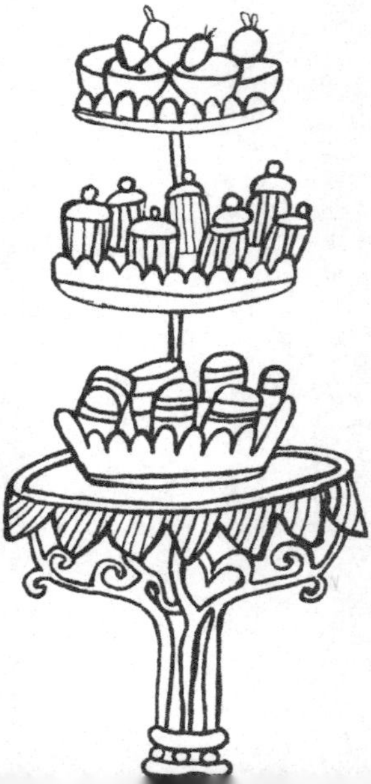

Cane sugar is our preferred option because it's always clearly marked on labels and we know what we're getting. Beet sugar is never clearly marked. Have you noticed that on the package of refined sugars, such as brown, granulated or confectioners it doesn't label the source of the sugar, whereas when it's cane sugar it's always proudly displayed? We can't say why, but what we do know is that on the labelling of 'sugar', manufacturers can include more than sixty different sweeteners derived, not only from cane or beet but also from many other sources, so we strongly recommend that you stick to the clearly marked cane sugar.

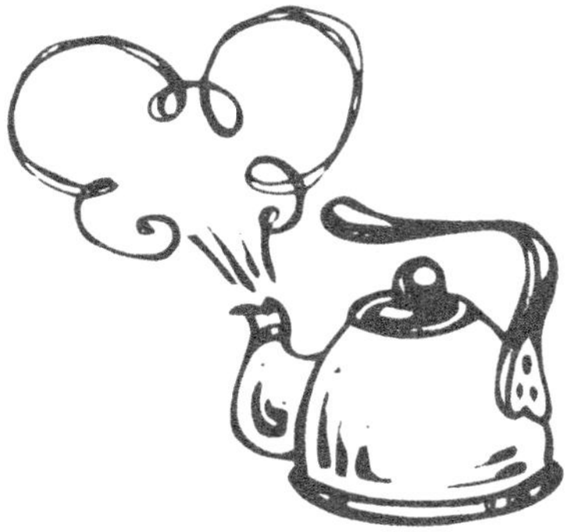

Artificial sweeteners are extremely bad for our bodies. People use them because they want to lose weight and yet the reality is just the opposite – it's the alternative sugars which promote weight gain. So be aware that they're sold under different labels: acesulfame K, aspartame, neotame, sucralose, saccharin, sodium cyclamate, to name a few. These sweeteners need to be digested before the body can absorb them. Other alternative sugars such as Stevia, corn syrup and Agave syrup are extracted from plants and also need to be digested.

So, why are artificial sweeteners and alternative sugars bad? For a start, they don't replace the need for sugar or glucose in the body and can potentially harm your liver and nervous system, rather than offering any benefit.

The body doesn't understand the difference between sugars, so when we have drinks with sugars that mimic cane sugar, they need to be digested. However, our bodies assume it's absorbable and doesn't prepare for digestion, which in turn can cause damage to the liver by contributing to fat storage and inflammation which can lead to liver enlargement. When the liver becomes fatty, inflamed or damaged, it doesn't function well. Its ability to burn excess fat and cholesterol is reduced, contributing to fatty deposits and weight gain. Studies have shown that sweetened beverages are associated with Type 2 diabetes. Why is this? Because all the diet and non-diet beverages are sweetened with alternative sugars.

Our liver helps to break down every single thing we put into our body and has an important role in digesting and absorbing the nutrients in food properly. So, when you're buying drinks, read the labels of soft drinks and sodas carefully and you'll notice that they contain 'sweeteners' rather than sugar, and especially not cane sugar. We should only sweeten beverages with cane sugar, which is kind to our liver. The only drink we've found containing exclusively cane sugar is the Mexican Coca Cola which is sold in the US. We love this drink! We don't drink too much cola, but as a treat, it's a favourite.

We can't say that sugar is the culprit behind obesity, but it's what is in the food that we eat that makes us fat, not the sugar itself.

In summary, to follow our Before 2 diet, after two in the afternoon, you can have drinks with sugar, but it should only be cane sugar as this won't restart the digestive process.

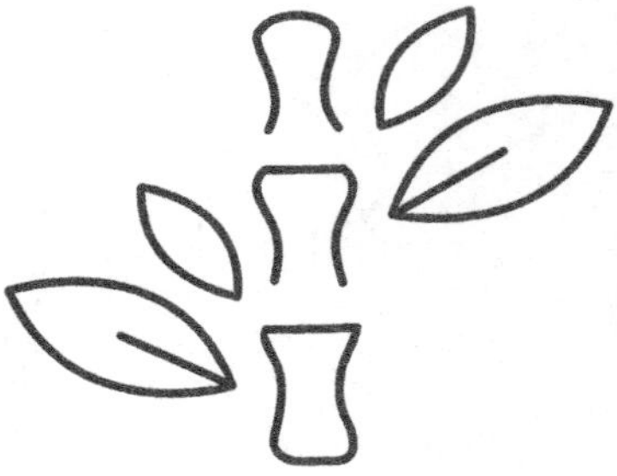

White Sugar or Brown Sugar?

It's useful to understand the different types of sugar currently on the market. It's assumed that brown sugar is more nutritional than white. Raw sugar comes from sugarcane, and at first, is only slightly brown. It becomes a dark brown colour when it's mixed with molasses. Manufacturers of sugar will bleach it to remove the molasses which makes the sugar white.

The truth is, they're not that different in terms of nutritional value. The molasses in brown sugar do contain minerals, but since they're in minute amounts, they don't bring any health benefit to the body.

The choice between white sugar and brown sugar is a matter of personal preference – as long as it's cane sugar, it's fine. You may notice that the labelling of white sugar in most countries doesn't explain what the source of the sugar is, because on most labels it's no longer sugarcane, but a mixture of different varieties.

To clarify, white sugar is good for you as long as it's clearly labelled as cane sugar.

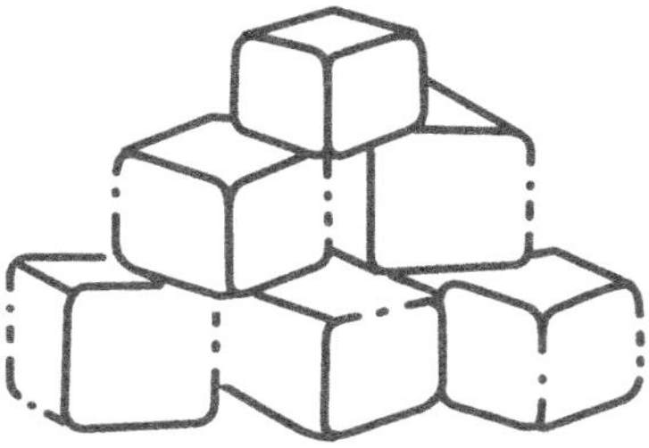

Muscovado Sugar

This is a variety of unrefined cane sugar where the molasses aren't removed. It comes in dark and light varieties and has a wet sticky, sandy texture, and a rich flavour. It's often used in baking to give a richer taste to cakes.

Turbinado Sugar

Turbinado is another type of minimally refined raw cane sugar. It has a caramel flavour and is commonly used to sweeten beverages, and can also be used in baking.

Demerara Sugar

Demerara sugar is a variety of raw cane sugar that's minimally refined with a caramel colour and flavour. It's used to sweeten drinks such as tea and coffee and is used in baking. Demerara sugar is not always made with cane sugar, but the best one to buy is where it's labelled: 'Made with 100% cane sugar.'

IN CONCLUSION

Ensure you buy only cane sugar for sweetening your drinks

Our energy and well-being will benefit from consuming some sugar

Cane sugar can be consumed without fear in desserts, drinks and food until 2 p.m. and the rest of the day in tea, coffee or any drinks

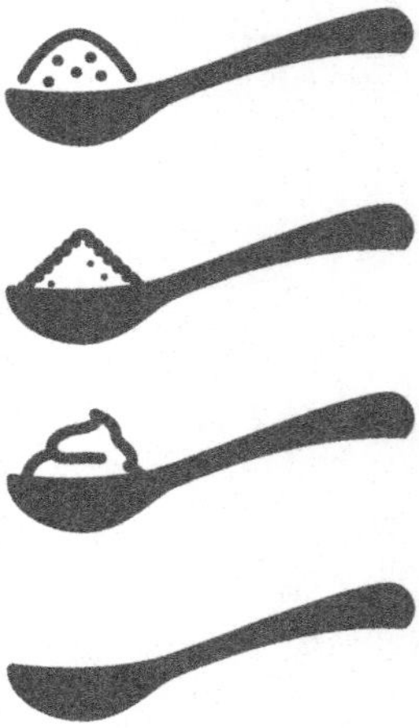

chapter nine

Pass the Salt

CHAPTER NINE

Pass the Salt

Salt is essential for the body. It controls the feeling of thirst and is a vital component of perspiration and tears. It's always been an important ingredient of our health, and is, in fact, indispensable to life, yet, surprisingly, the body cannot produce salt – it has to rely on our regular intake with the food we eat.

The kidneys also need salt to function properly. Our body regulates salt levels carefully to prevent them getting too high or too low. The sodium in the salt controls the formation of urine and the kidneys are responsible for retaining or expelling sodium in the urine depending on our body's requirements. That's why we should maintain adequate levels of salt in our blood.

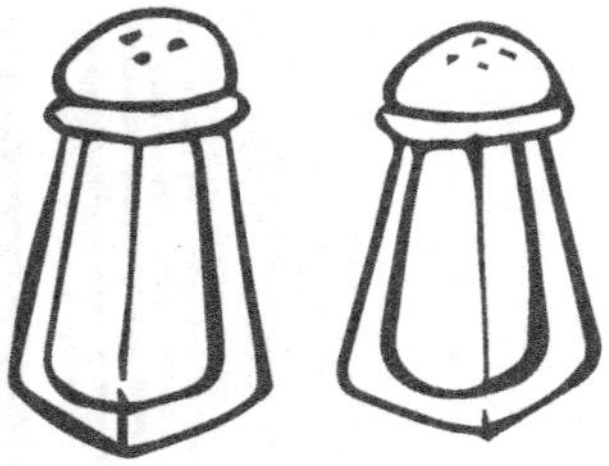

Amongst the condiments found for the preparation of food, salt is one of the oldest, dating back to around 2700 B.C. There are two main forms of salt:

Rock salt
mined from the earth

Sea salt
harvested from the ocean

Salt is so necessary that humans have always had to search their environment to fulfil this need, and some animals, notably elephants, will walk for hundreds of miles to hidden salt caves which their ancestors used in prehistoric times. In the vicinity of the caves lie countless carcasses of dead elephants, giving rise to the theory that salt was a sacred food for them and a place akin to a spiritual ancestral home.

American pioneers crossing over mountains while seeking a new life had to follow the trails created by generations of wild animals to lead them to salt sources. The Egyptians extracted their salt from the river Nile while the Chinese collected salt from the lakes during the dry season when the water evaporated. Apart from being an indispensable item of food, salt also allowed them – and still does, of course – to preserve meat for consumption in the bleak winter months. Salt draws the bacteria-causing moisture out of foods, drying what remains, and making it possible to store meat for long periods without needing refrigeration.

While it's possible to develop a taste for salt that exceeds our actual needs, our drive to eat salty foods reflects a real need to maintain an adequate body salt content.

Salt is made from two elements: sodium and chloride. The body relies on sodium for a variety of functions, including keeping blood pressure under control and the transmission of nerve impulses. It dissolves in the body's fluids, notably our blood, and supports thyroid function, and is needed for digestion and brain function to help with clarity of thinking.

Where did this idea that salt is bad stem from? Many years of scientific research have failed to prove any benefits arising from a low-salt diet. The evidence is weak and new studies have found that, at the recommended intake, salt may have a beneficial role in our health.

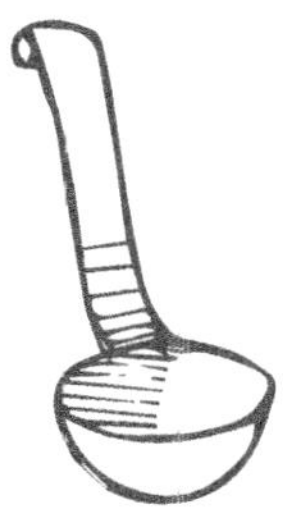

The human craving for salt isn't just a bad habit – it appears to be a biological need as fundamental and as powerful as thirst. The real question is: What amount is too little and what is too much? One thing we know is that the need for salt varies with each individual. The recommended daily amount of salt is six grams per day which is the equivalent of one teaspoon. Some people may need more or less. NB: children between one to three years only need two grams a day. Consulting your doctor on the individual intake is recommended.

Salt vs Sodium

Sodium is a mineral that's found in salt which is also added to processed food in much higher quantities than you find in salt, such as tinned food and ready-meals. Therefore, processed ready-to-eat foods are not a healthy choice for a nutritious diet. This is another reason why it's important to eat fresh food that you can prepare yourself, so you know exactly what's going into your food.

We suggest that salt should only be eaten in the morning or early afternoon, before 2 p.m., as anything we eat in the morning will be digested easily and won't harm your body.

To follow the Before 2 diet, you cannot take drinks with salt after 2 p.m. because salt needs to be digested, as it's also considered to be a food. So those Margarita cocktails will have to be drunk before 2 p.m.

Salt doesn't just make our food taste delicious, it's more than a seasoning... it's essential for life.

- Only eat salt before 2 p.m.
- Salt makes you hungry and will enhance your appetite for enjoying a large meal in the morning or at lunchtime.

- **Table Salt**
  Created by heating natural salt to the point where beneficial compounds are destroyed. It's also bleached. We don't recommend it.

- **Sea Salt**
  Contains a small amount of natural iodine which is a good thing. It's typically much less refined than table salt.

- **Pink Himalayan Rock Salt**
  Comes from ancient seabeds in the Himalayan mountains. The pink colour is derived from its rich iron content. This salt is rich in minerals, containing all eighty-four essential trace elements required by our body. It's our favourite salt.

- **Other salts such as Grey Salt**
  For every forty kilos of grey salt produced, one and a half kilos of delicate *Fleur de Sel* is harvested. These light, flaky salts are good quality. In terms of health, they are simply highly-priced sea salts with a delicate flavour.

Buy your ingredients fresh and cook your own meals. Avoid processed food as much as possible

We need to eat a certain amount of salt with our food as the body cannot produce it itself

Salt does not make you fat

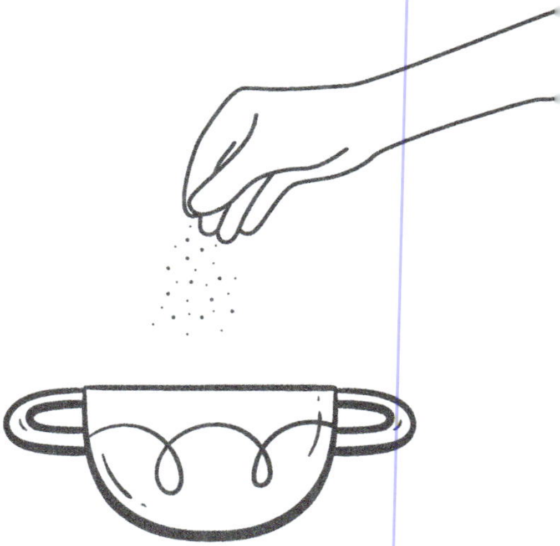

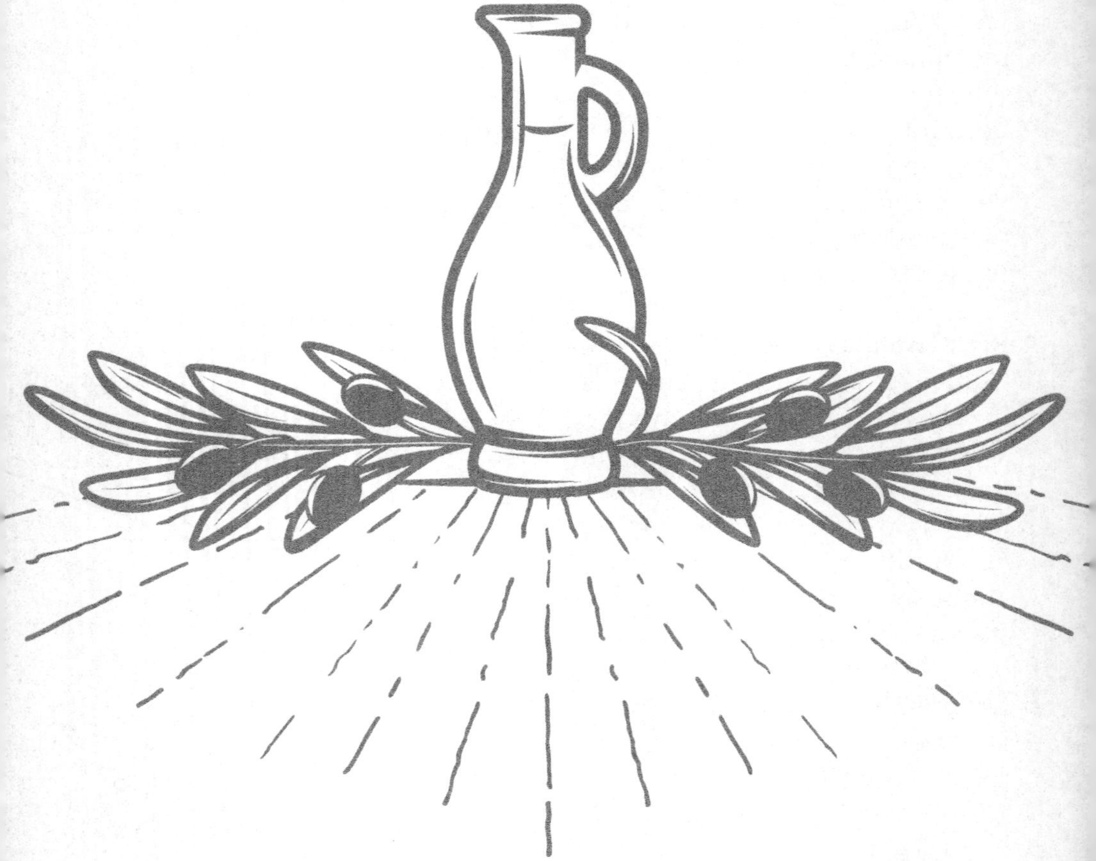

chapter ten

Good Fats vs Bad Fats

CHAPTER TEN

Good Fats vs Bad Fats

For decades, nutritionists and doctors have preached that a low-fat diet is the key to losing weight, managing cholesterol and preventing a variety of health problems. But while many have significantly reduced their fat intake, obesity has more than doubled. How could this happen? We believe it all comes down to the time that you eat as well as the good or bad fats we consume.

- **Good fats are essential for physical and emotional health.** The good fats – saturated fats and unsaturated fats – protect your heart and support overall health.

- **Bad fats such as artificial fats or trans fats, increase cholesterol and the risk of heart attacks and other diseases.** They're also associated with a high risk of developing Type 2 Diabetes and they can make us fat too.

Trans Fats

Let's delve a bit further into this subject that has baffled scientists and often left the general public even more confused.

When we talk about 'bad fats', it's usually in reference to 'trans fats' and their role in our digestion. Trans fats were the first man-made fat to become part of our food supply more than a century ago when an experiment intended for making soap took place. Hydrogen was added to cottonseed oil and as a result, the oil looked like lard. This suggested that hydrogenated oil or trans fats could be an inexpensive substitute for butter and lard in our food, and it also increased its shelf life. At the time, switching from butter or lard to a product made from a healthy vegetable oil seemed like a good idea, especially for losing weight – suddenly, trans fats became widely produced from vegetable oils and replaced natural fats in many types of food.

So, why did trans fats become so popular if they have such bad effects on our health? Well, it took many years of study and it wasn't until the late 1990s, that this type of fat became a serious health concern and manufacturers were required to list trans fats on food labels.

These trans fats are extremely difficult to digest as they don't break down like natural fats during the digestive process —so, it's like eating plastic— they don't have any nutritional value and they clog up our arteries.

A TV documentary in 2010 showed how a London sewer had been clogged up with hydrogenated fats or trans fats; the blockage caused sewer overflows. To be removed, this fat had to be hacked away with shovels, high-pressure water jets, and powerful vacuum units. This is exactly what happens to our arteries when we consume artificial fats.

Sadly, for many years natural fats have been wrongly blamed for the damage caused by trans fats. Most restaurants use trans fats in their deep fat fryers because it doesn't have to be changed as often as natural oils and fats. Trans fats are also found in many products on supermarket shelves such as fried and baked products e.g. crisps, biscuits, cakes, croissants, frozen pizzas, pastries, margarine and bread. They're also heavily used to make simulated meat, for example, vegetarian sausages and burgers.

A mandate from the *New York City Board of Health* in 2007 confirmed how bad trans fats are and restricted their use in 22,000 restaurants. Our advice is to avoid these fats as much as possible.

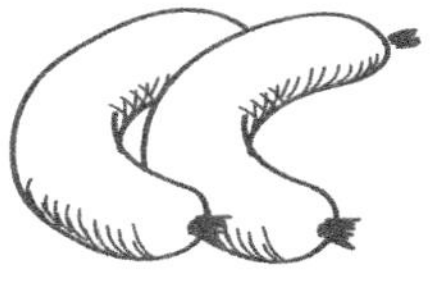

Interesterified (IE) Fat

If this wasn't enough to be concerned about, more recently, a newer type of artificial fat appeared, called Interesterified (IE) fat. This was introduced as a replacement for trans fats and is taking its place in a large range of products, particularly spreads, baked goods and confectionery.

IE fat was developed by artificially altering the molecules of oils to modify their melting point. This process increases its role in food production, allowing the shelf life of food products to be extended. The effects of IE fat on the human body are not fully understood as few studies have been conducted. We don't know enough about these new fats, but we'd recommend avoiding products containing IE fats until more research has been done.

There's no legal requirement for food manufacturers to include IE fats on food labels. These would be found in products where modified oils are used and the labels will only list the name of such oils as soybean, rapeseed, palm, sunflower and so on.

Good fats and protein

Eating an adequate amount of good fats, saturated fats or animal fats is important for our health as well as unsaturated fats which are found in plants. These foods contain good fats which provide a source of stored energy and in turn give shape to our body, cushioning our skin, and acting as insulation, because they can be properly digested.

We're not delving into a separate chapter on protein, but suffice to say if you eat animal products like meat, fish, eggs, or dairy products daily, you're also getting the right amount of complete protein in your meals. Protein is the main building blocks of our body, for bones, muscles, cartilage, skin, and blood. Our body uses protein to build and repair tissue. It also helps supply the nutrients we need.

Good fats are one of the main components, present throughout the body. They also help the body to absorb vitamins and minerals. Certified Nutrition Specialist and personal trainer, Mike Geary, author of *The Truth About Six Pack Abs,* says: "Why did members of the Maasai of East Africa remain free from degenerative diseases on diets consisting of large quantities of raw whole milk, blood and meat?" The Maasai are an ethnic group of people living in East Africa who settled in Kenya and northern Tanzania. Traditional Maasai life revolves around their cattle which are their primary source of food. Two-thirds of their calories come from animal fat. They consume 600–2,000mg of cholesterol a day (the recommended intake being 300mg per day.) They maintain low blood pressure and cholesterol levels and have low rates of disease.

When it comes to meat, some people prefer it to be from grass-fed cows, others prefer the meat from corn and soy-fed cows. The term grass-fed isn't so clear as not all grass-fed cows graze outdoors. Depending on each country, cows, pigs and poultry are often fed with antibiotics and hormones: this is a much more important factor to avoid than the type of food animals eat. And when it comes to chicken and eggs, organic is the best choice and a priority before free-range – but organic free-range is by far preferable. For dairy products, the full fat is a much better choice – as long as you don't have lactose intolerance. The full fat in our milk is necessary in the stomach as it helps digest the rest of the milk. Natural fats don't make you fat.

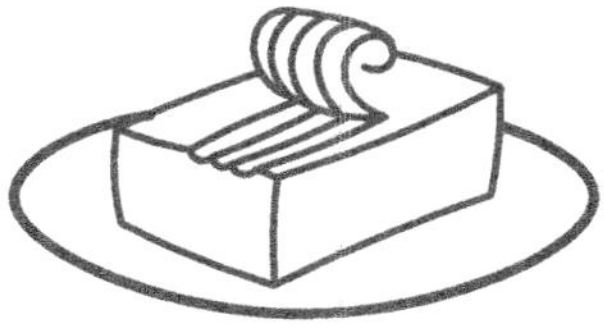

Vegetarian and Vegan

A common concern about vegetarian and vegan diets is that they might lack sufficient fat and protein, however, a well-planned diet can provide all the nutrients you need.

For vegetarians, dairy products and eggs are a good source of fat and protein.

Vegans can get their fat from vegetable oils such as olive oil and peanut oil, peanut butter, avocados, and nuts e.g. almonds, cashews, and peanuts.

Pulses and grains are particularly important for people who don't get protein from eating meat, fish or dairy products. Pulses such as lentils, kidney or black beans, quinoa and chickpeas are amongst the highest in protein.

Animal-based foods such as eggs, dairy, fish, and meat contain complete proteins while most plant foods are incomplete. For a complete protein, a food item must contain nine amino acids in equal amounts. When it's incomplete it means that certain amino acids are missing, but if you're vegan you can easily combine two or more foods to make up the complete protein. Rice and beans are a good example of a complete protein because the amino acids that are missing from beans are found in rice, and vice versa. Many other food combinations are also considered to be complete protein sources.

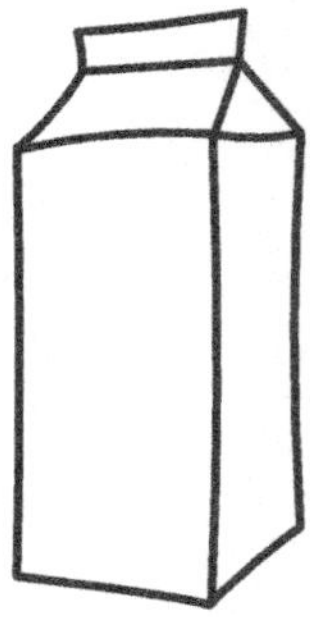

Oils

Oils that come from plants are called monounsaturated fats and are good for us, especially extra virgin olive oil, and peanut (groundnut) oil. Olive oil is better for salads and low heat frying as the smoke point is not as high as peanut oil which is good for high heat frying. An oil's smoke point is the stage when the oil starts burning and is an important thing to consider. If you heat an oil past its smoke point, it not only harms the taste of your food, but it becomes toxic to the body.

The liver cannot digest burnt oil or burnt butter. It's therefore important to avoid burning fats and oils. If you enjoy the taste of low heat frying with butter, the butter should always be mixed with a spoon of oil. Never fry with butter alone as it will burn.

To clarify, we recommend you use extra virgin olive oil and peanut (groundnut) oil for all your cooking, as other oils have a very low smoke point and may be extremely processed.

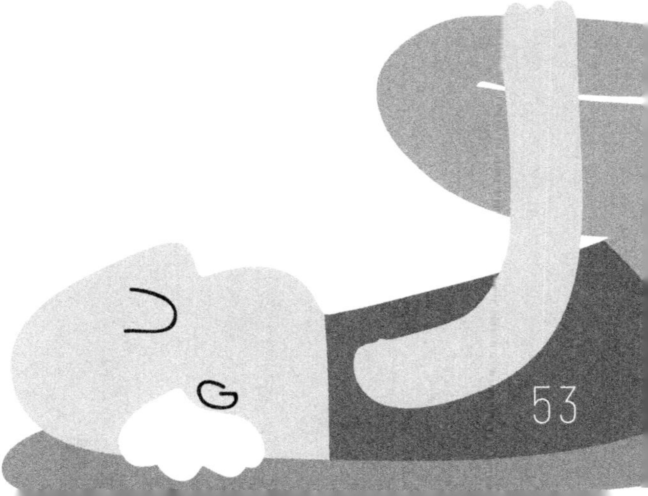

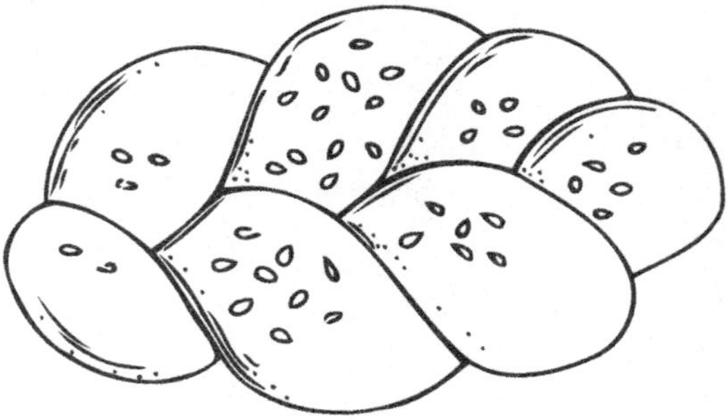

chapter eleven

Carbs

CHAPTER ELEVEN

Carbs

Many diet books these days carry a belief that starchy foods are the enemy and must be avoided at all costs. But as with so many assumptions about diet, food and digestion, the use of 'carbs' has simply had an undeserved bad press.

We believe our diet should always include a certain amount of carbs. Starch is the main source of energy for the human body and is found in bread, rice, potatoes and pasta.

However, there is some information suggesting that carbs should be reduced or removed from your diet if you don't use up much energy, such as doing a sedentary job in an office. This is a myth. Calories aren't only used when you engage in physical activities; the body is constantly using energy to keep the heart pumping and your digestive system functioning as well as regulating breathing, managing hormones, and maintaining body temperature.

Taking carbs out of our diet means that the body would have to use fat and muscle tissue to provide glucose for the brain. This would cause us to lose weight, but it would be an unhealthy way of doing so. We would lose muscle and the necessary healthy fats needed, consequently making us look aged before our time with dry, lined skin and less muscle tone. Without carbs, the body will then switch to using protein as a fuel source and this can lead to symptoms such as dizziness, shaky hands, lack of concentration and feeling cold.

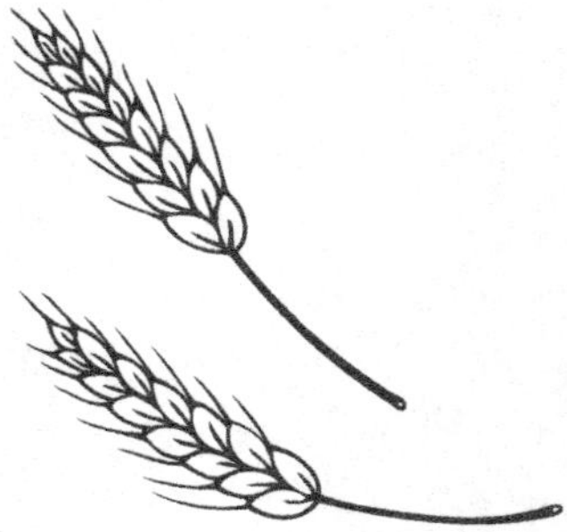

The idea that starchy food is fattening leaves people confused about their importance in maintaining a healthy weight. We can tell you that it won't make you fat when it's eaten early in the day. Starches are highly nutritious and valuable to a healthy diet and they contain calcium, iron and B vitamins. Starchy vegetables are also easily incorporated into our food consumption, making good side dishes for our meals. Carbs are also an incredibly flexible food source suitable for meat-eaters, vegetarians and vegans. Potatoes, rice, pasta and couscous are also a great accompaniment to meat, vegetables or salad.

Bread is another starchy food which has been a staple of human food and has been eaten worldwide for thousands of years, made from flour and water.

There are so many varieties of bread available in our modern society, including sourdough, sweet bread, soda bread, baguette, pita bread and many more. However, the bread that we buy in supermarkets today is not the healthiest. It contains so many unnatural additives, made with huge quantities of yeast and no fermentation time at all. And this is why many people are affected by allergies or have complaints about bloating. There are many independent bakeries or bakeries within supermarkets which make fresh bread. Making homemade bread is also a great solution and is fun and easy. Making no-knead bread at home it's so quick and simple, that even children can make it. The same dough can also be used to make a good homemade pizza base.

All these starchy foods can be enjoyed as part of a healthy diet. Just eat them before 2 p.m.

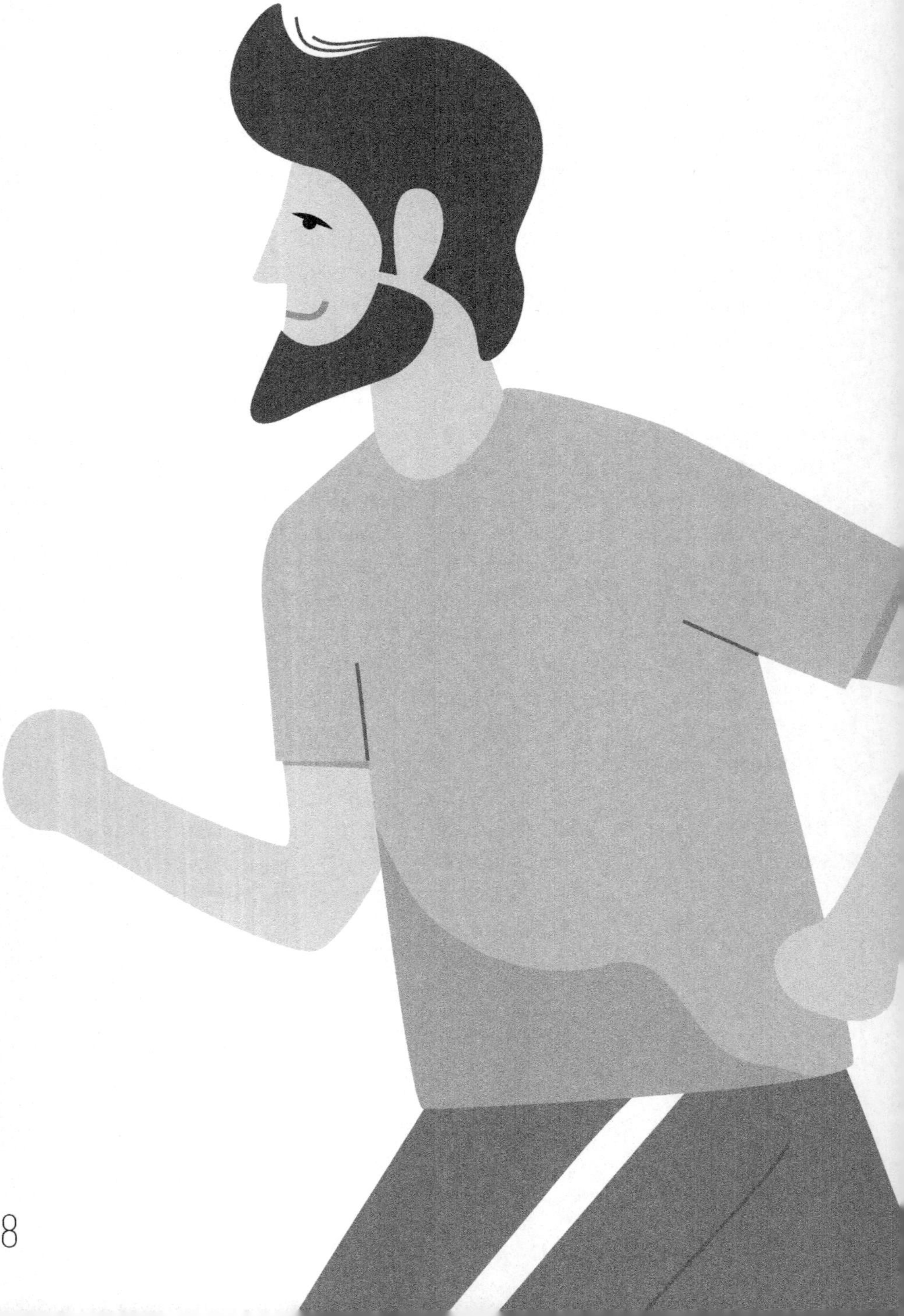

chapter twelve

Vitamins – Synthetic vs Natural

CHAPTER TWELVE

Vitamins – Synthetic vs Natural

The discovery of vitamins back in 1912 was a major scientific achievement in the understanding of health. The previous belief was that only four nutritional factors were essential: proteins, carbohydrates, fats, and minerals. Now vitamins were added, causing more excitement than all the rest put together. This breakthrough led chemists to isolate these vitamins by figuring out their chemical structure, and they were able to develop ways to create synthetic supplements.

Our understanding of vitamins continues to evolve from that time. Most people believe that if vitamins aren't effective, at least they are safe. However, many studies have revealed a series of side effects that can be harmful to our health.

Natural nutrients
These are obtained from food.

Synthetic nutrients
Supplements. These are usually made artificially in an industrial process.

Vitamins and mineral supplements should come with a 'handle with care' label as they don't absorb in our digestive system in the same way food does. The majority of supplements available in health shops are made artificially. These include vitamins, minerals, antioxidants, amino acids, and many others. They can be found in the shape of pills, powders and liquid, and they've been designed to mimic the natural nutrients in food. The production process of these synthetic nutrients vary hugely to the way plants and animals create them and this includes supplements that claim to be made from 'natural' ingredients.

When we eat a meal, the food is not in a condition that our bodies can use as nourishment. It must first be changed into smaller molecules before the nutrients can be absorbed into the bloodstream and carried to the cells. When we take a supplement, it's a highly concentrated dose that we'd never get from food alone. As a result, those vitamins may not be fully absorbed by the body, causing unpleasant side effects and potentially damaging our health.

Mineral pills, for example, can cause tooth staining, increased urination, stomach bleeding and an irregular heart rate.

Vitamin C is needed daily as it's not retained by the body like other vitamins. Two large oranges can provide our full daily Vitamin C requirement, and you can also source this from many other fruit and vegetables. If you come down with a virus such as a cold or flu, Vitamin C can also strengthen your immune system in fighting it off. Although taking Vitamin C in excess when you already have a diet rich in fruit and vegetables could cause stomach upsets and diarrhoea, destroy red blood cells and cause kidney stones. An excess of Vitamin A can cause hair loss and blurred vision, and too much Vitamin D can cause nausea and diarrhoea.

These are some of the side effects that we know of and we suspect there are many others. Mostly, however, these supplements are filtered straight out of the body and therefore don't contribute any nutritional value. And if you're already absorbing a wide range of natural nutrients through your diet, taking extra supplements can cause us to exceed the recommended daily intake.

Synthetic nutrients are no replacement for a healthy and balanced diet. A lack of vitamins and minerals are due to either a poor diet – in which case you need to eat a wider variety of food – or your body may not be fully absorbing the nutrients from the food you eat.
When we eat in the evening, we'll have either incomplete digestion or zero digestion of any food eaten. If we don't digest our food fully, the body cannot absorb the nutrients it needs. If, on the other hand, we eat our food earlier in the day, when the digestive system is working at its best, the digestion will be complete and the absorption of the nutrients into the bloodstream will be highly effective.

To conclude, a varied diet generally provides more than enough of each vitamin and mineral, and our bodies will use nutrients best when taken in natural food such as a selection of fruit, vegetables, meat, dairy, pulses and cereals.

Here are a few of the guidelines we need to follow if we're serious about achieving a balanced intake of vitamins and nutrients:

Eating all the nutrients we need from our food is the best recipe for a healthy life.

A variety of food sources contain all the vitamins and minerals needed for good health. Supplements aren't necessary.

Digestion of our food and absorption of nutrients work best when we eat before 2 p.m.

Fortified foods

In some fortified foods, vitamins or minerals are added that wouldn't normally be there. Other fortified foods are enriched with nutrients because these were lost during processing and are then added back in the form of synthetic supplements. For example, skimmed milk is fortified with vitamin D, cereals are commonly fortified with B vitamins, and calcium may be added to fruit juices. Many fortified foods currently available contain levels of vitamins that aren't appropriate for younger children and they are at risk of overdosing.

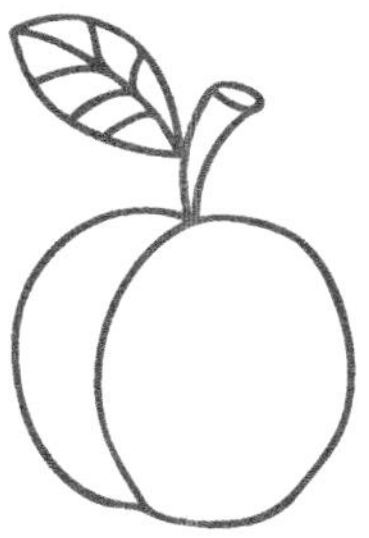

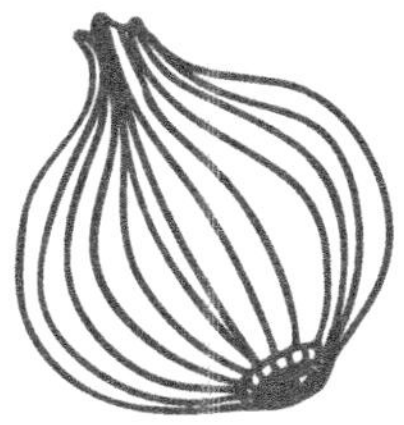

Taking these added supplements won't improve a poor diet. For most of us, the best solution is to eat as varied a diet as possible, combined with other healthy lifestyle changes.

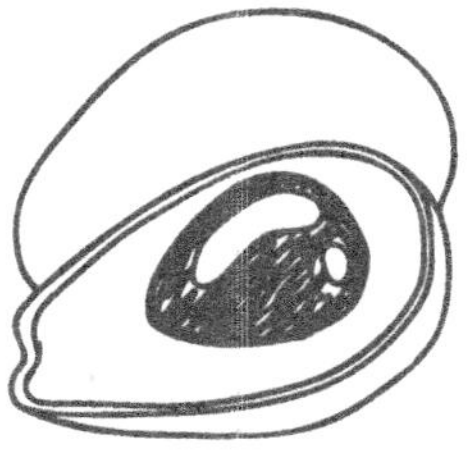

Here's a list of nutrients that are crucial for good health, together with the best food sources for each. This shows how simple and easy it is to have the correct nutrients in our food.

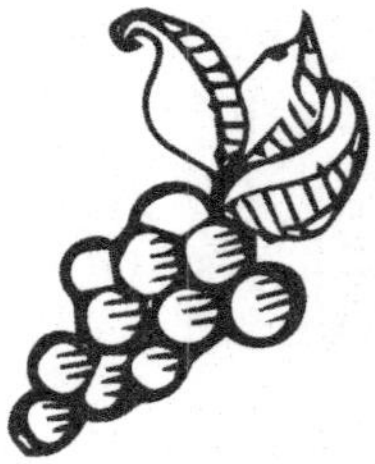

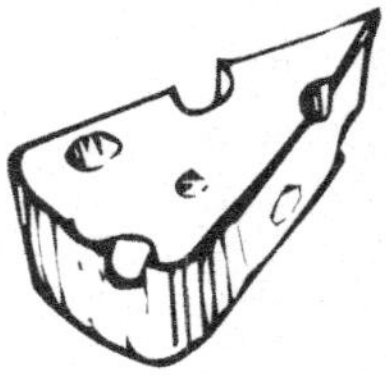

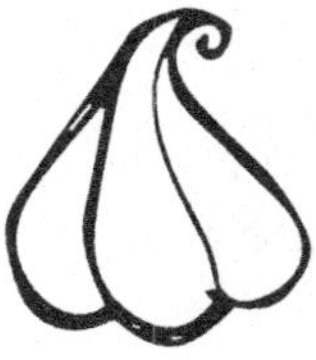

Nutrient	Source
Vitamin A	Eggs, whole milk, cream, cod liver oil, broccoli, spinach and most dark green leafy vegetables
Vitamin B	Eggs, whole milk, cheese, meat, nuts, avocados, bananas, bread, citrus fruits, beans, lentils
Vitamin C	Oranges, lemons, grapefruit, limes, guava, kiwi and vegetables such as broccoli, cauliflower and brussel sprouts
Vitamin D	Salmon, most fatty fish, cod liver oil, egg yolks, liver, whole milk, cheese, mushrooms. Spending time in the sun is also a good way of getting your daily dose of Vitamin D
Vitamin E	Nuts such as almonds, peanuts and hazelnuts, sunflower seeds, avocado, spinach, broccoli
Vitamin K	Kale, spinach, brussel sprouts, broccoli, cauliflower, cabbage, whole milk, cream
Folic Acid	Dark leafy greens, asparagus, broccoli, citrus fruits, beans, peas, nuts, cauliflower, beets, corn
Calcium	Dairy products such as whole milk, cheese, yoghurt, cream, beans, lentils
Iron	Clams, oysters, liver, spinach, pumpkin seeds, beans, lentils
Zinc	Seafood, spinach, cashews, beans, bread, cocoa
Chromium	Fresh vegetables, herbs, grains

conclusion

A New You, a New Start

CONCLUSION

A New You, a New Start

To start this diet, make a decision which requires replacing old eating habits with new ones. Everything we do every single day involves making a choice, whether it's deciding what to have for lunch, whether to say yes to a social invitation, applying for a new job or buying a house. A single decision can make a huge difference in your life.

When we align ourselves with the way our bodies are designed, eating early, then fasting after 2 p.m. for the rest of the day and going to bed early most nights, we can see amazing changes. The result will be gradual weight loss, noticeable almost immediately, and revived energy levels you haven't experienced since you were a teenager – a new vitality that's reflected in your eyes, your posture and your smile, along with a more positive attitude to life. After a while, you'll understand how every cell in the body is closely tied to our circadian rhythms. Every aspect of our body has a time for everything and the time to eat is early in the day. You'll also see that going against our natural rhythms requires much more effort, causing our body to work less efficiently.

Remember to Drink

Remember to drink plenty of liquid with your food, and also remember, your meals don't have to be low fat. Eat the good fats and even eat those delicious dishes you thought would make you fat such as spaghetti carbonara or sausages and mashed potatoes because eating our meals at the correct time of the day turns all the food into energy. And remember to finish your meal with a delicious dessert or you may crave something sweet later when you see your friends eating pancakes, cakes, ice creams and chocolates.

Are you Ready?

So, are you ready to embark on this voyage to health, weight loss, and a sexy, slender physique? Stick to the Before 2 diet and as promised you should notice the difference within one week. Live life in harmony with your natural circadian rhythms and see what happens. Give it a try, and remember that you can break this diet for special occasions, such as Christmas, a wedding, or an office party. And then wait for that moment when you meet an old friend who exclaims, "Wow, you look fabulous... what have you done?"

Like a butterfly emerging from its chrysalis, a beautiful new you will emerge. Take a chance... it'll be worth it!

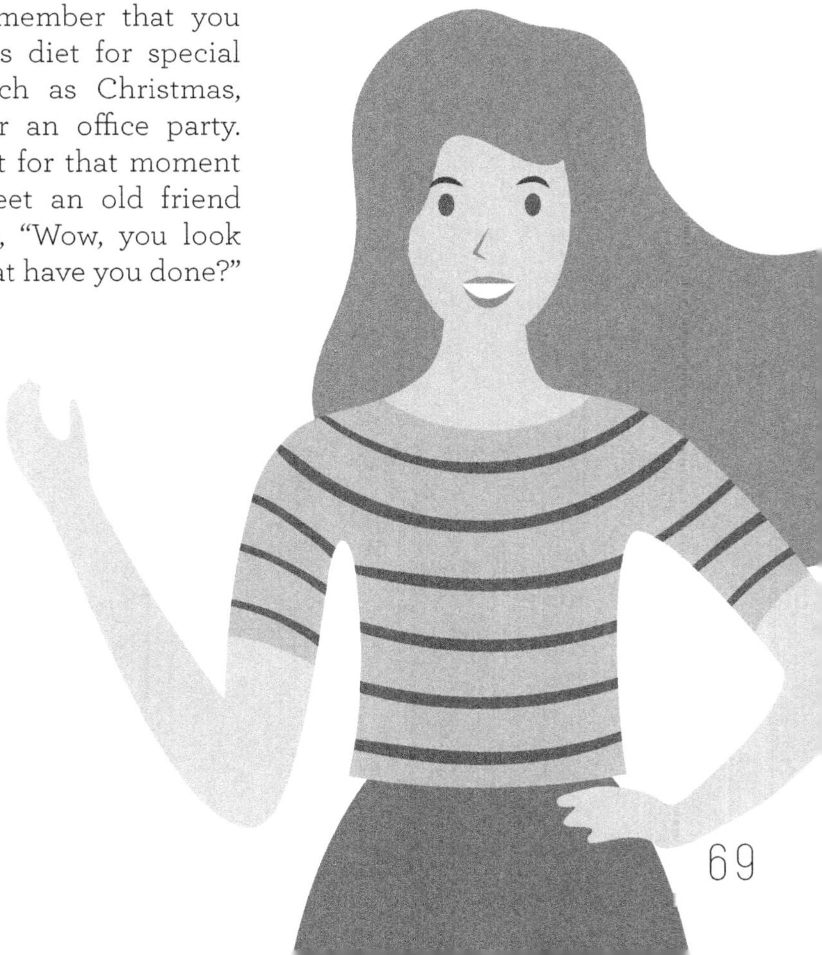

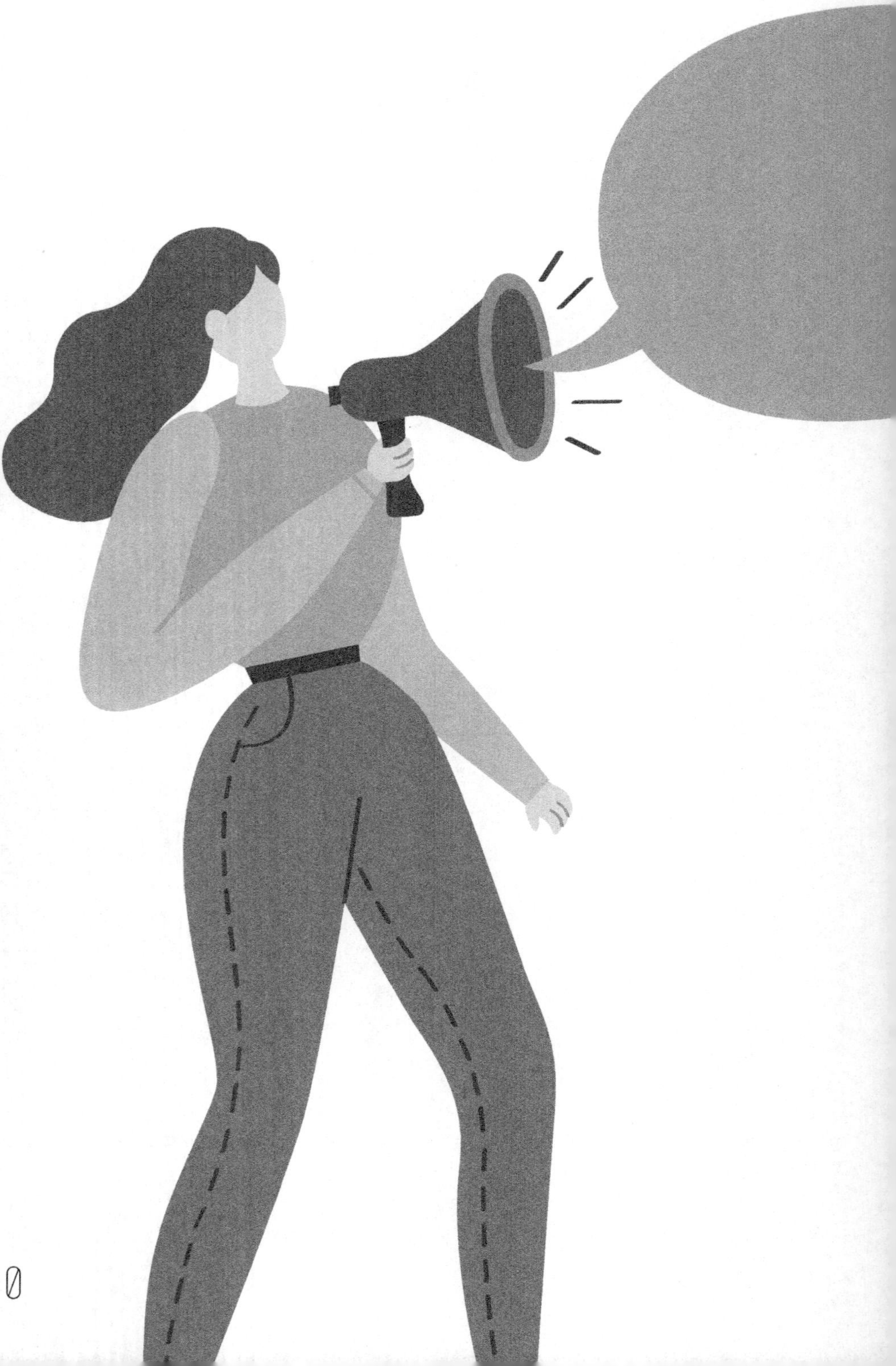

testimonials

TESTIMONIALS

"I'm sixty-three and have never succeeded with any diet until now. I work from home spending long hours on the phone in front of my computer. Most days I'd eat snacks all day with copious amounts of coffee. Then I'd have a big meal at 8.30 p.m. I don't get ill often but I developed an unpleasant acid reflux and it took me several weeks to realise it wasn't going away, so my doctor prescribed a daily tablet.

Although it did the trick for a while, I still felt uncomfortable. I also needed to lose weight and wasn't sleeping well. When I met Diana at a book launch and she explained the simplicity of Before 2, eating anything you want and as much as you want until 2 p.m., I was excited as I love food! It really was a life-changer. I eat as much as I always have before 2 p.m. and because of the fasting from the afternoon, I drink much less coffee. The biggest surprise is that three months into the diet, I didn't feel hungry at night anymore. I've lost the excess weight, my skin is clearer, I sleep better than I've done for years and I have no more heartburn! I feel rejuvenated and alive!"

Sherry Humphreys, based in Brighton, UK, letting agent

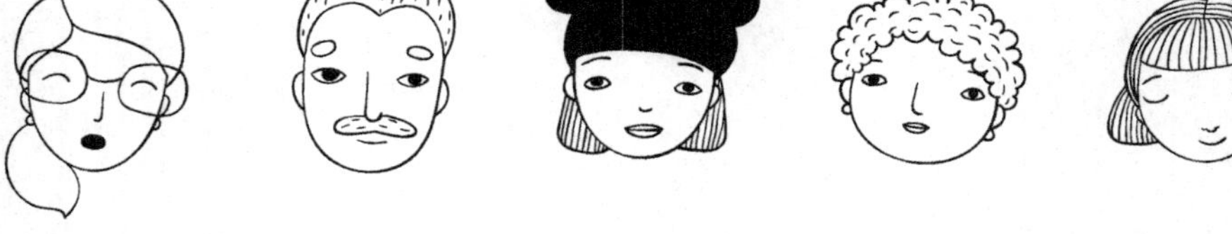

"Before 2 helped me immensely. I started it by wanting to shed a few pounds and soon noticed it was also alleviating my digestive issues. For many years I'd been suffering from a hiatal hernia and acid reflux. After six months I stopped taking my stomach medication which wasn't helping much and had long term side effects. I've followed the Before 2 way of eating for three years now and, although I'm slim, I also feel healthy and enjoy my life. I greatly appreciate Diana's contribution because this is not just a weight loss diet but rather a new way of living"

Tatiana Brooke, based in Miami, USA, court interpreter

"I thought I knew everything about food until I went on the 'Before 2' diet. Now I know that I will never go back to my old ways of eating which were accompanied by constant struggles with weight and feeling sluggish. I've not only lost weight, but I have a lot more energy, better muscle tone and I feel healthier than ever before. This is the only way of eating that makes sense. I can eat everything I desire and it's sustainable as I don't feel I'm missing out."

Angus Macleod, based in West Sussex, UK, holistic medicine therapist

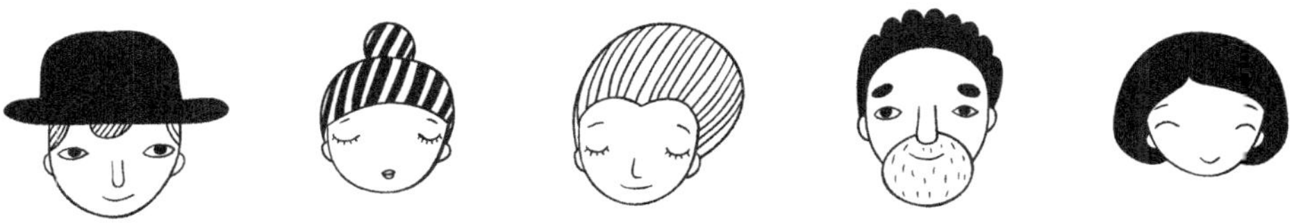

TESTIMONIALS

"I'm a chef and love food. As a result, I eat more than most people. I get to prepare the most delicious dishes for my clients, but naturally, I started putting on weight. I met with Diana in a café in Buenos Aires when she was visiting her family there. I hadn't seen her for many years and was surprised to see her looking so slim and lovely. She told me about her eating plan and that I wouldn't need to eat less to lose a few pounds, only that I needed to eat meals before 2 p.m. I wasn't certain that such a small change could make a difference to my weight, but I needed to get healthier, so I decided to give it a try. After two weeks on this diet, I'd already lost six kilos as well as feeling lighter and more energetic. I still enjoy all kinds of food, such as pizza, pastas, fish, meats and cakes, including full-fat dishes, for breakfast and lunch. I have since slimmed down to my normal size 12 and have a renewed zest for life."

Lidia Lebon lives in Buenos Aires, Argentina, works in catering

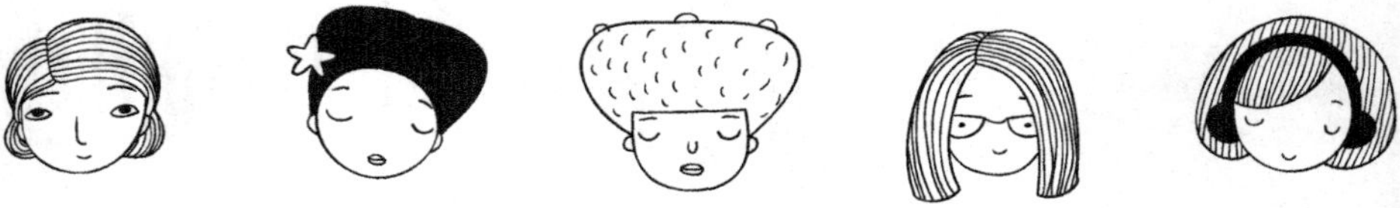

"I've been following the Before 2 eating plan for many years and it's completely transformed my health. If I do eat later in the day, my energy takes a nosedive and I have a restless night's sleep. It was a little difficult in the beginning, especially for my children but after a couple of weeks, they weren't remotely hungry in the evening. And even now at seventy I still have the energy to lead a full and active life thanks to eating before 2 p.m."

Nina Anne Fordham lives in Brighton, UK, works as an auxiliary nurse and craniosacral therapist

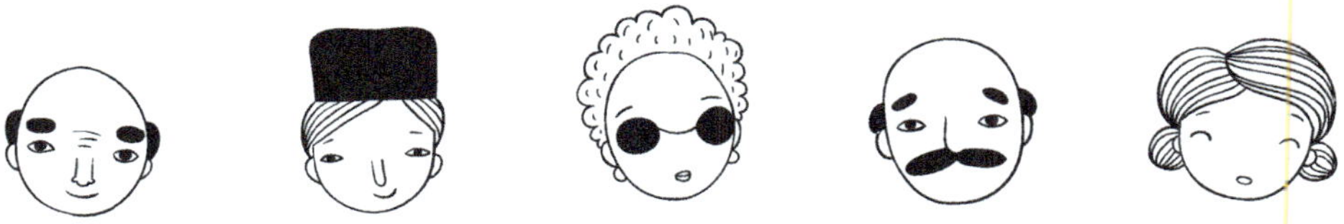

references

1. Matthew Walker. *The Joe Rogan Experience #1109*
YouTube, April 25, 2018. **www.youtube.com/watch?v=pwaWilO_Pig**

2. Garaulet, Marta, Ordovás, Jose. *Chronobiology and Obesity. NewYork. Springer (2013).*

3. Garaulet, M., Gómez-Abellán, P., Alburquerque-Béjar, J. et al.Timing of food intake predicts weight loss effectiveness. *International Journal of Obesity 37, 604–611 (2013).* **https://doi.org/10.1038/ijo.2012.229**

4. Walker, Matthew. *Why We Sleep. Great Britain. Penguin Books (2018).* **p. 340**

5. Michael Geary. *The Truth about Six Pack Abs. Vervante (2006)* **p. 35**

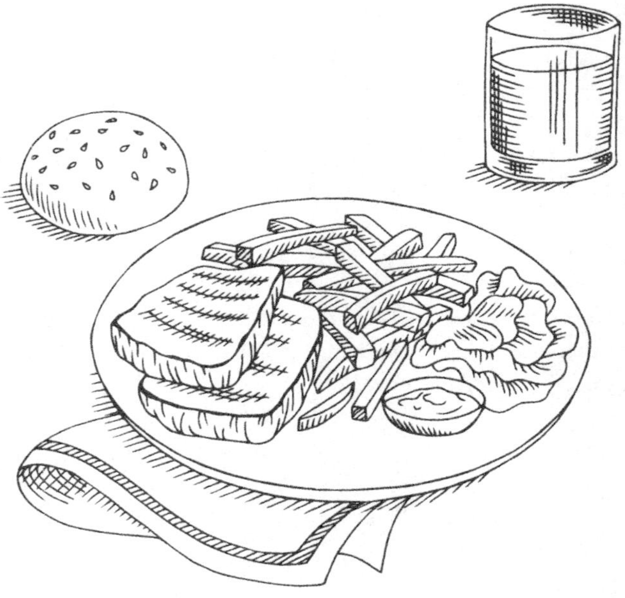

notes

Space for Reflection

In this space we invite you to create your own experience with Before 2. Make notes, check your measurements and so on.

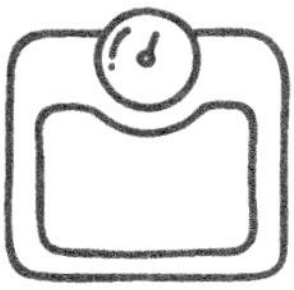

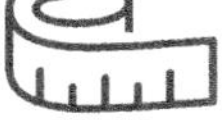

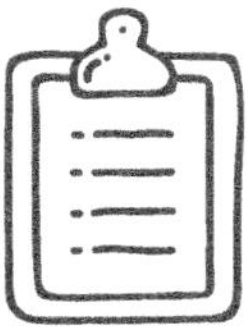

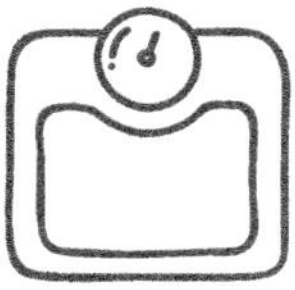

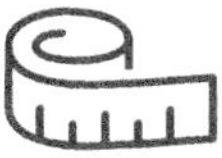

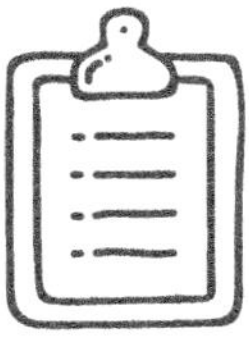

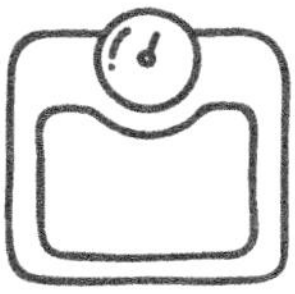

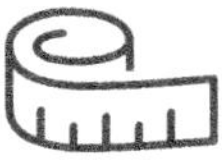

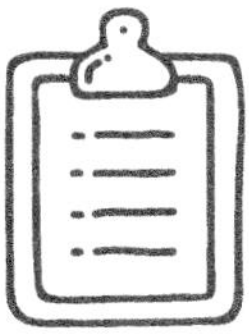

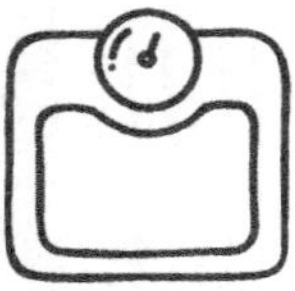

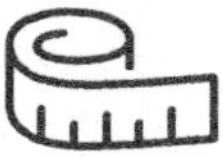

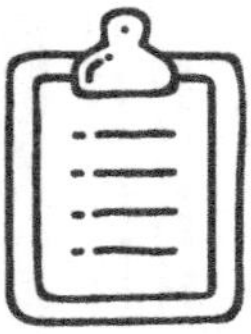

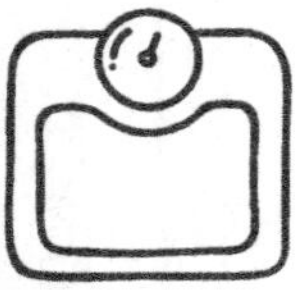

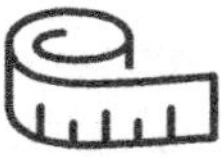

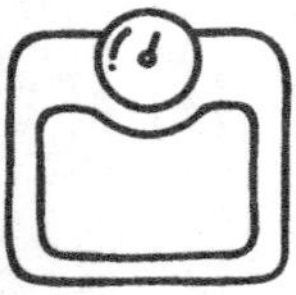

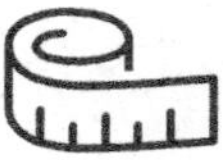

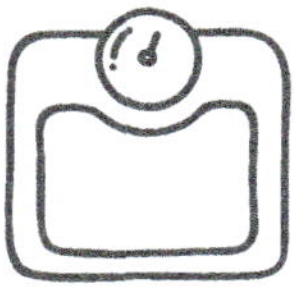

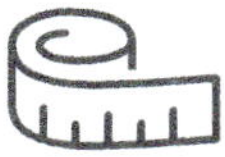

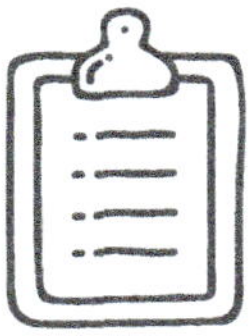

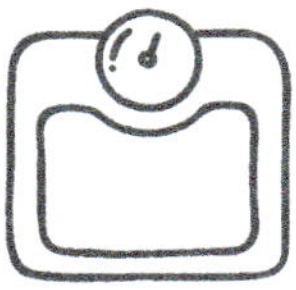

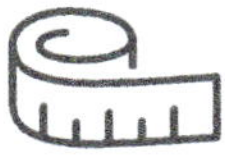

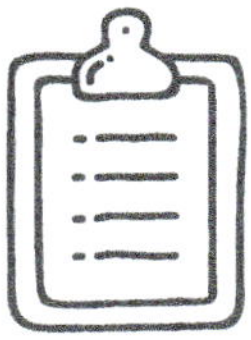

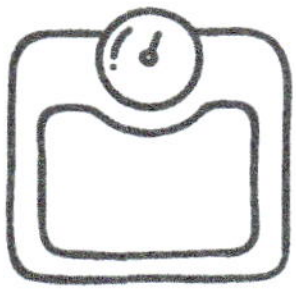

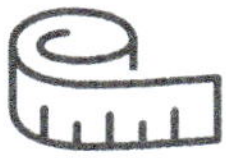

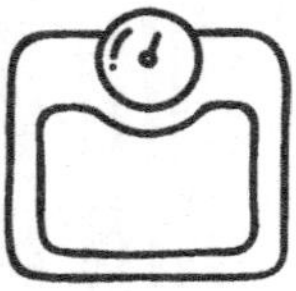

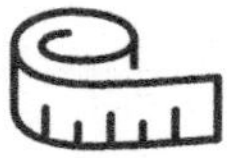

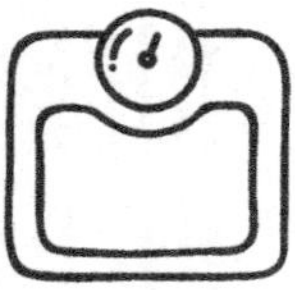

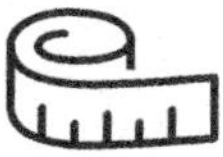

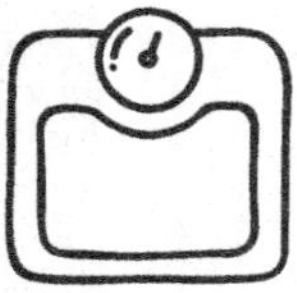

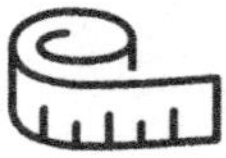

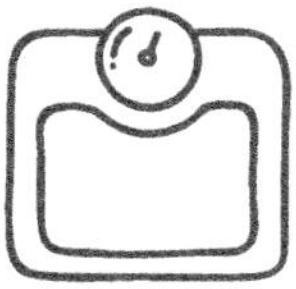

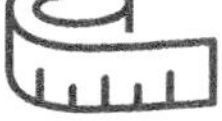

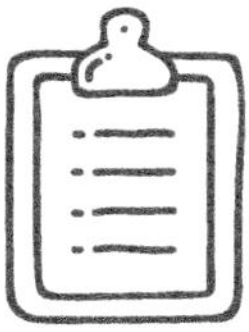

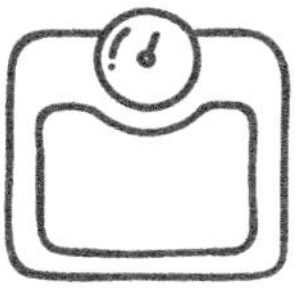

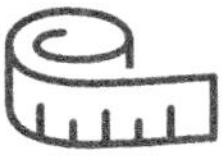

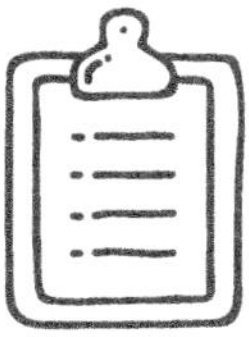

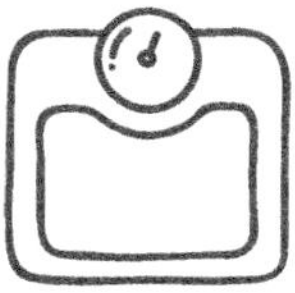

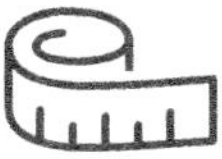

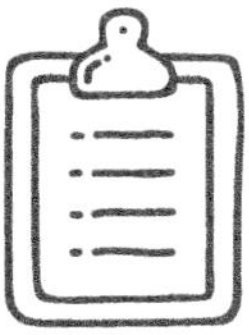

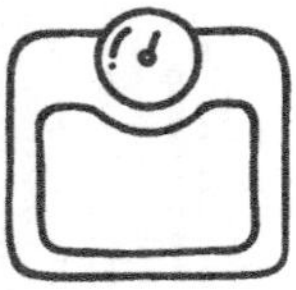

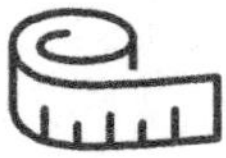

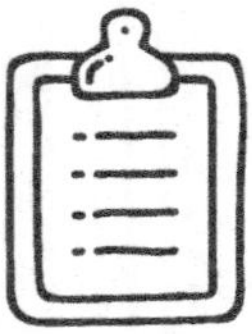

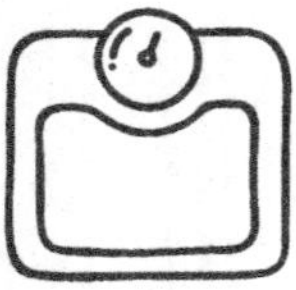

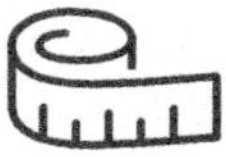

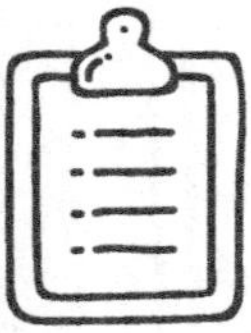

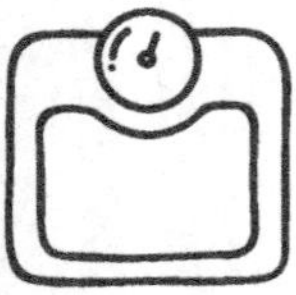

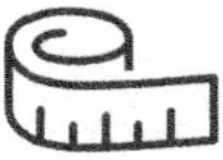

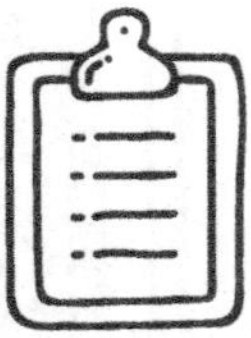

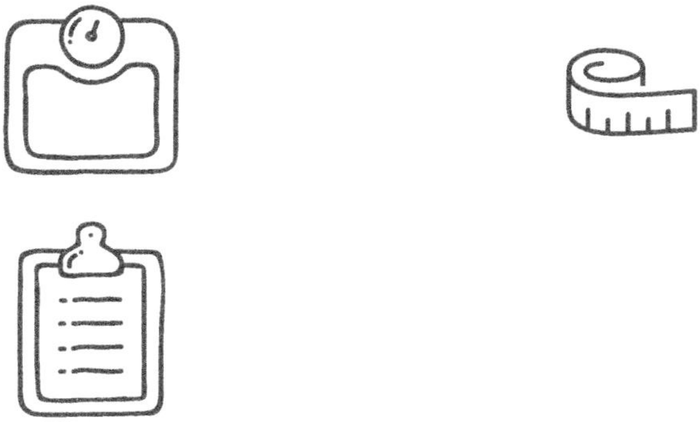

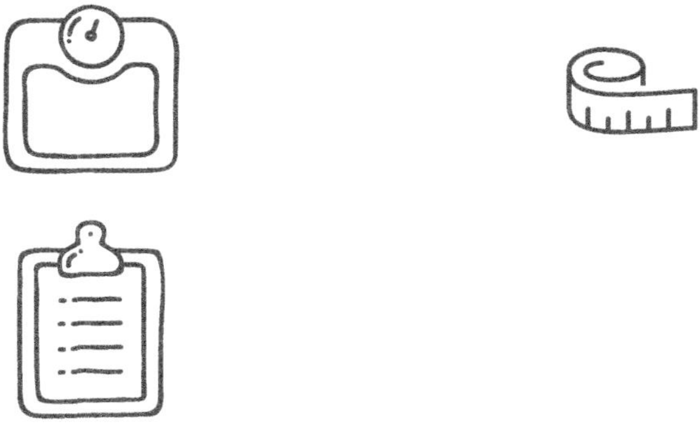

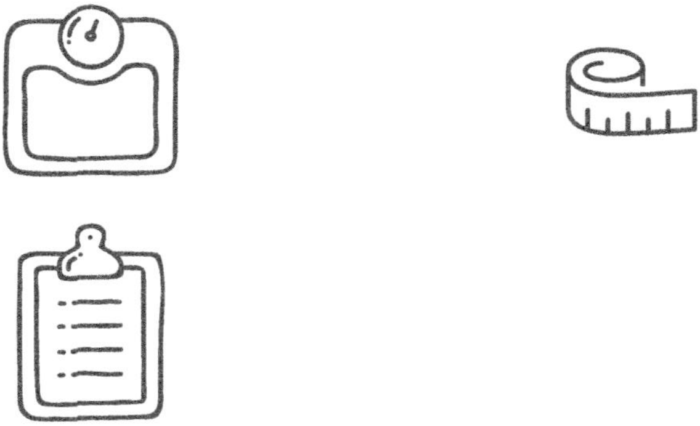

Printed in Great Britain
by Amazon

21176527R00059